A
(somewhat irreverent)

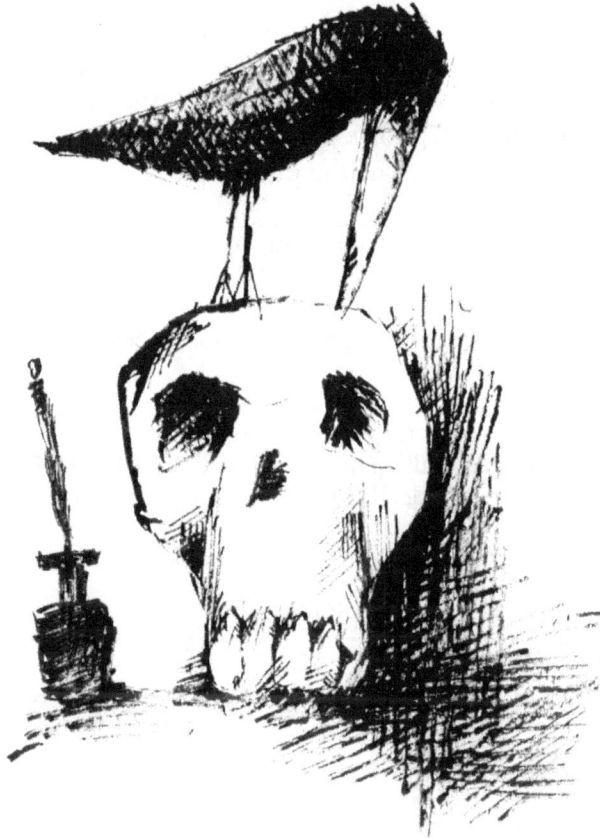

INTRODUCTION TO PHILOSOPHY
for
MEDICAL STUDENTS
and other busy people

Niall McLaren, M.D.

Future Psychiatry Press

A (Somewhat Irreverent) Introduction to Philosophy for Medical Students and Other Busy People
Copyright © 2012 by Niall McLaren. All Rights Reserved.

Cover picture and cover design by Michal Splho
www.FuturePsychiatry.com

Library of Congress Cataloging-in-Publication Data

McLaren, Niall, 1947-
  A (somewhat irreverent) introduction to philosophy for medical students and other busy people / Niall McLaren.
     p. cm.
  Includes bibliographical references (p.   ) and index.
  ISBN 978-1-61599-156-3 (pbk. : alk. paper) -- ISBN 978-1-61599-155-6 (ebook)
  1. Philosophy--Introductions. I. Title. II. Title: Introduction to philosophy for medical students and other busy people.
  BD21.M336 2012
  100--dc23
                         2012009521

Distributed by: Baker & Taylor, Ingram Book Group, Quality Books

Future Psychiatry Press is an imprint of
Loving Healing Press
5145 Pontiac Trail
Ann Arbor, MI 48105
USA

http://www.LovingHealing.com or
info@LovingHealing.com
Fax +1 734 663 6861

CONTENTS

Also by Niall McLaren, M.D.

Humanizing Madness: Psychiatry and the Cognitive Neurosciences (2008)
Humanizing Psychiatry: The Biocognitive Model (2009)
Humanizing Psychiatrists: Toward A Humane Psychiatry (2010)

From Future Psychiatry Press

Introduction

Since my books have been published, I have had anxious emails from students around the world complaining that there are too many big words in them. One in particular startled me: "Why do you use foreign languages?" he moaned. "Nobody knows them nowadays. It's hard enough reading this stuff in English, let alone in French." Actually, the quote he mentioned was Latin but his complaint was valid. I studied medicine and psychiatry with two dictionaries on my desk, one English and the other the old Dorland's Medical Dictionary. I still have both of them and use them most days. The reason we have so many big words is just because they are precise: yesterday, I had to check on the difference between 'misconstrued' and 'misconceived.' There is a difference, because we use different words to denote the differences we discern. In Western countries, we have only one word for rice; Indonesian has three and Thai seems to have about a dozen. I'm told Mexicans have about 50 words for chili, but don't laugh: look at all the words we have for different types of beer.

Most of the words students have trouble with are not taught in medicine; they come from the discipline called philosophy. Unfortunately for medical students and other busy people, if you do not use a word regularly, it is often difficult to remember exactly what it means. This can be troublesome as words are tools; they allow us to explore the full meaning of a concept and understand why it means just that and nothing else. It is more of a problem in psychiatry than in other fields because the concepts we are relying on are often hidden. Even when they are dragged out into the full light of day, they are slippery notions that are difficult to pin down. Partly, this is because medical people are not used to thinking in terms of abstract concepts (there isn't a lot of abstraction in a microscope slide) and partly because the concepts themselves may not be clearly understood anyway.

So the difficult words are our (sometimes feeble) attempts to isolate and define the precise meaning of an even more difficult concept. These lectures are my suggestion as to how students (and don't forget, we are all students) can look at the types of concepts used in psychiatry and similar fields. I am not a philosopher; I have studied philosophy at undergraduate level (and enjoyed every moment of it) and have focused on a number of areas as they relate to the work I do but I do not have the breadth and depth of specialist background a professional philosopher needs. My work is about mental disorder so I don't take too much notice of the concept, say, of a just war, or of the further reaches of the philosophy of mathematics. If you want to know more about them, you'll have to do what I did, and go back to school.

Where do we start? Probably the first word to define is philosophy itself. Like so many important words, it comes from the Greeks: *philos-*, love of, and *-sophist*, a wordsmith or person who uses words to argue a point. Sophists were wandering teachers who taught the sons of the upper classes how to reason and argue their case, which was important for people who tried to govern themselves by reason rather than by force. However, the sophists got a bit of a bad reputation because very often, they turned into smart alecs, using clever wordplay to defeat their opponents rather than winning their case by reason. The modern equivalent would be lawyers who use semantic loopholes in the law to defeat its purpose, or politicians who use a fog of words to evade taking responsibility or to conceal their intention. And here we have your first important lesson in philosophy: *declare your prejudices*. "Oh," you may say, "I'm a very reasonable person. I don't actually have any prejudices." OK, but that's your second lesson: like it or not, everybody has prejudices. The very words you use are loaded with meaning and you need to understand that your listeners are entitled to apply their own meanings to words, or to find hidden consequences in your statements. So my prejudice is this: I believe very firmly in the notion of *noblesse oblige*, which is French for the idea that people in positions of power have a burden of responsibility to do the right thing by their juniors. So a person with a good education or with high verbal facility is under a duty to ensure that he doesn't use his education or his clever tongue to put one over people who didn't have his advantages in life. There's another prejudice (or habit, there's not a lot of difference): I use male pronouns. The reason I do this will become clear as we go along.

Getting back to the modern sophists, there are far too many people these days using their education to pull the wool over the eyes of the general public. This is especially bitter as every smart alec in the world has been educated more or less completely at public expense (*alec*, I just found in my dictionary, is slang for a stupid person or a fool; a smart alec is therefore a smart or educated fool). In medicine and other specialized areas, it is very easy to use your education to take advantage of people, so easy that, sometimes, it is difficult to be sure they have made their own decision and not been swayed by the awesome figure talking to them. In psychiatry, which deals in the most difficult areas –and the most frightening – we have a very real burden of responsibility to speak clearly in words our audience will understand, and to be sure that we fully understand the hidden consequences of everything we say to them. As my work shows, this is almost never the case. Psychiatrists have not analyzed their belief systems or their modes of action, but they don't suffer from their own neglect, only the disadvantaged do. We'll come back to this point.

The second major point is that there is no such thing as philosophy. Oh, what a terrible thing to say, but it's true. If you want to build a bridge, there is a particular body of information you have to learn before you start digging your holes. If you want to defend a man in court, there is a body of knowledge called The Law that you have to know in case they string him up. The same is true of surgeons cutting people open but, about philosophy, there is no agreement. The subject matter of philosophy is this: any complex issue, without limit. You can be a philosopher of poetry if you wish, or of the death penalty, or of beauty or religion. The best we can say is that a philosopher is a person who philosophizes; that is, he approaches complex questions from a particular point of view. The point of view is to examine critically the unstated abstract notions hidden behind the facts he is looking at or underlying the explanations he offers, or buried deep in the language he is using. In order to do this, he needs a set of methods and principles (tools, if you must) that allow (or at least don't hinder too much) the process of dissecting an idea or situation to find its basic concepts and, eventually, its justification.

So, a person who sets up shop as a philosopher of the death sentence will not be much concerned with statistics of how many people get the chop, who, where, how and why (although these may be important to confirm a general principle he has discovered). Instead, he will be looking abstractly at the notion of what is the best method of execution (should it be humane or grotesque, private or in public, etc) in order to achieve its goal, whatever that is. He will also look at who should get it under what circumstances and, ultimately, whether we have the right to put somebody to death. Needless to say, all these hidden questions will be intimately interwoven and very, very highly charged, so a person who decides to be a philosopher of the death penalty will actually have a very difficult job. He can also be sure of one thing: whatever he decides, most people will disagree violently with his conclusions. He should also be aware that if people do agree with him, they probably had a hidden agenda anyway. Finally, he should remain mindful of all the philosophers who have gained their understanding of the meaning of the death penalty from first-hand experience.

This brings us to the next purpose in philosophizing: to convince people, to sway them, change their minds and make them see things from a different point of view but NOT to convert them. A philosopher is never a preacher. His job is to analyze the question from every possible point of view and reach a conclusion that is dictated by the material (and not by his prejudices, politics, money etc). If the world agrees with him, all well and good; he will probably be invited to give lectures in luxury resorts in exotic locations to groups of sleek, well-heeled people who nod approvingly at everything he says before rushing out to lunch to continue doing exactly what they were doing before (making money, drinking, gambling with other people's lives, procuring... the usual stuff the wealthy get up to). But if the world doesn't agree with him (far and away the most likely outcome), the best he can hope for is a job in a small university teaching little groups of irreverent students while slaving over his next paper that might just get him tenure.

If, however, he is lucky and can mumble French while smoking foul black cigarettes, and is equipped with a cosmic disregard for the niceties of society, he may become a media superstar and will earn heaps of money from dictating a stream of books that convince people who want to be convinced that what they have always believed is right. That, however, is extremely rare so, boys and girls, here is your next lesson: philosophy is not a winner. If you want to make money, or get ahead, or be well-known or popular or well-dressed, look elsewhere. On your introductory day at university, you should hurry past philosophy to the economics department, or do an MBA, or even become an engineer or a plastic surgeon, but don't feel sorry for the bearded, bespectacled and uninspiring philosopher standing forlornly by the hand-written sign saying "This way to the secrets of the universe." If he really had any secrets, they wouldn't be in a loose-leaf file.

There is, however, an advantage in being philosophically inclined in medicine or similar fields: if you don't like social chit-chat, or parties, or dinners or that sort of nice thing, learn a few big words and get some interesting angles on the stem cell debate. You won't be invited back. The message is simple: most of the time, most people don't want to be challenged on most topics, especially topics they regard as important. Most people want their prejudices reinforced. The last thing they want is to have them stripped bare and shown to be brainless, self-contradictory gibberish. People want security, they need it; they crave it just because humans fear uncertainty. We do not like to have our treasured beliefs overturned; they are treasured because they make us feel good. We need our prejudices and deepest beliefs: they are *amicus certus in re incerta,* a certain friend in uncertain times, and the less secure we are in ourselves, the more we need firm, unwavering beliefs to bolster ourselves. Straight away, you see a psychological element intruding in what ought to be a rational area.

Unfortunately, this is a lesson I never learned at university and it cost me dearly. I arrived at an unknown provincial university in the mid-sixties, from a tiny country town, the first person in my entire family to have completed high school. I had a head full of notions of university as a place of liberal scholarship, notions which would have been out of date even in the thirties, when the books I had been reading were written. As it was, I had never even seen the university when I started there, and had never spoken to a graduate (students didn't speak to teachers in those days unless apologizing). I thought everybody would be friendly, helpful and keen to learn by brave self-criticism. How very wrong I was. It turned out that, in respect of open-mindedness, academics were far worse than the genial farmers, shopkeepers and fishermen I had grown up with. Fortunately for me, that was the era of Vietnam so it was easy enough to find people who were opposed to the status quo, except I soon learned they were interested in criticism, but not in *self*-criticism. As a result, my time at medical school was not happy but I leapt into psychiatry thinking this would welcome free-thinking. Once again, I was mistaken. The professors were rigid, convinced, and vengeful. They didn't want anybody questioning them. Their lectures were exercises in narcissism, not adventures in enquiry. They were not interested in new information, they were angered by it and, as I soon learned, they had ways of dealing with people who made them angry.

After I graduated as a psychiatrist, I started the long process of teaching myself but it was not easy. At the advanced age of 34yrs, I was accepted as a joint candidate for a PhD in the department of philosophy and the department of psychiatry at my university but it didn't go well. The psychiatrists were manifestly not interested as they saw no point in anybody questioning the received view. The philosophers were much more fun, they liked the idea of having a psychiatrist in their classes but one thing I learned very quickly: despite my years in medical school, my degrees and my status (chief psychiatrist in a veterans' hospital), I didn't know how to think. I was in a class with teenage students: already, they could go to the heart of a matter much quicker than I could. Over the next year or two, I caught up with them but then I learned something else: in my rush to catch up with the philosophers, I had lost contact with my psychiatric colleagues. They were no longer interested in anything I had to say. A couple of times, I was actually prevented from finishing lectures, and soon I wasn't invited to give any more. I was shepherded away from medical students and my name somehow slipped off the list of supervisors for trainees (residents).

Was this planned? Did they huddle together and say, "We don't like what this bloke is saying, so let's kick him out of our sandpit"? I don't think so. There was simply an unspoken agreement that the interests of the medical students, the trainees and of the other psychiatrists were best served by everybody learning the truth about psychiatry, and they alone knew the truth.

The message for medical students is this: it might be amusing to poke fun at your professor's dopey ideas, but don't expect any gratitude from him. Thrusting young lecturers don't get up the greasy academic pole by criticizing the Grand Old Men (and women); they get ahead by memorizing the party line and parroting it at every turn. So if you want to get ahead in psychiatry, or medicine, or anything, throw this book away now. If a large office with elegant carpets and gracious potted palms is your goal, if you like conferences and research grants and degrees and gowns, dump this book in the nearest bin (or press delete). Find a get-ahead professor, sit at his feet, tell him what he wants to hear and you too will soon be sliding up that well-known pole. But whatever you do, don't scare him by asking him to look critically at his beliefs. He will hit back, that much is guaranteed.

* * *

To summarize, humans have beliefs. Beliefs are very influential in controlling behavior. Not all beliefs are known explicitly to the individual, some beliefs are implicit. Implicit (unconscious) beliefs are real and effective. An implicit belief is more likely to be irrational, or contradictory, or just plain wrong than one that has been explicitly learned and is clearly understood by its owner. Most people do not like having their implicit beliefs questioned because it makes them look stupid. Humans do not like being made to look stupid and will get even.

Beliefs do not exist in isolation. Every belief we hold has to jostle inside our heads for shelf space with a lot of other beliefs. Eventually, they all sit on top of each other like hats in a shop window display: individual beliefs are, you could say, "nested" in a larger belief structure. We would like to think that each little belief hangs logically and coherently from a hook on a larger belief, and that from another, on and on until we come to the Really Big Hook from which your entire belief structure hangs. The Really Big Hook might be God, or it might be Survival of the Fittest or, if there are still any Marxists out there, it would be Historical Determinism, something like that. That one big hook constitutes your **ontology**, your fundamental belief system concerning the nature of things as they are. If you hold a particular religious belief system, then your ontology is **supernatural**: humans consist of an animal body and a supernatural soul. In most religious systems, the supernatural entities can intervene in daily life without causing the universe to melt down. If you deny a religious basis to the universe, you hold to one or other form of a **materialist** ontology (words in **bold** are defined in the glossary at the end of this book).

Because there is no direct evidence about the nature of the universe, questions of this type go beyond facts. They are called **metaphysics**, which just means 'beyond physics.' Some people would like to think that we can get away from metaphysical questions because they can never be answered firmly but that only shows how dull and boring they are. For philosophers, questions that can never be answered firmly, that go on and on, seemingly forever, are the most interesting type. The most deceptive trap for a scientist is when he is talking about a question he thinks is **empirical** (i.e. one that can be solved by additional facts; or a belief which can be changed by further evidence) but it is, in fact, metaphysical. Physicists and other bright people are now awake to this sort of problem because they tinker with the nature of reality and time and matter and energy, so they are never short of inquisitive philosophers peering over their shoulders. The worst examples of metaphysical questions being dealt with as though they were empirical is in, guess what? That's right, psychiatry. In the later chapters, we'll spend a lot more time on this point.

There is no such thing as philosophy. The day job of the philosopher is to look critically at any complex issue to make sure it is not just a case of prejudice or stupidity, or metaphysics masquerading as empirical science (or vice versa). Philosophy is not a science, it is not something that can be memorized and regurgitated during exams: it is all about ideas. It is a mode of enquiry, an attitude or general approach to examining complex issues. During their training, philosophers learn some standard methods of questioning and, from studying the history of ideas, they recognize many famous errors that people have made in the past. They learn to group ideas and how ideas relate to each other but mostly, they learn to enquire and examine and tease ideas apart until they find the full set of beliefs from ontology down to microcosm. The whole point of philosophy is to stand back and look critically at the question from a distance, comparing different ideas in a field. Generally, this is identified by adding the prefix meta- to the field. So we get metamathematics, meaning a general analysis of what mathematicians do, without getting bogged down in individual sums. Metahistory is an interesting one, it compares different theories of the nature of historical progress. Is history decided by Great Men or is it, for example, the outcome of unseen social forces. This is usually called historiography, but it's the same thing. Metapsychology compares different theories of psychology, but that is usually known as either the philosophy of mind or the philosophy of psychology. People often claim that Freud wrote a metapsychology, but he didn't. He wrote a metaphysical psychology, which is something completely different – and wrong.

One of the techniques philosophers can use is **logic**. Logic is not a science but it is more or less the verbal equivalent of mathematics. Maths is about the relationships between quantities; logic is about the relationships between ideas. Logic is the study of valid inference or, if you prefer, the study of consistent beliefs. It uses particular forms to work out how two ideas are related, whether they are validly related or whether they are inconsistent. Logic is not much concerned with the real world; it is more about possibility than reality. So logicians talk about "possible worlds," like: Could there be a world in which the Australian cricket team always beats their mortal enemies, the English cricket team? Yes, there could. There is nothing in the notion of always walloping the Poms (rather unpleasant slang for English gentlemen) that breaches any logical rules. Could there be a world in which Mick Jagger sang a song that Mick Jagger didn't write? Yes, there could. Could there be a world in which Mick Jagger wrote a song that Mick Jagger didn't write? No, that would be impossible. Could there be a world in which Elvis is still alive? Yes, that is a logical possibility. Could there be a world in which he is both dead and alive? Well, that depends on how you define the word 'or,' as in "Elvis is either dead or he is alive." Some definitions of 'or' are inclusive ("Would you prefer tea or coffee?" "Thanks, I'll have both.") while some are exclusive ("He is either married or single") meaning he can't be both at once (being married and acting single doesn't count).

Logic is about relationships so it blurs across to mathematics and to computer sciences, since computers are essentially logic machines. I firmly believe that logic should be part of every high school course, just as maths and English are. It's that basic to life. If you can't tell when somebody is pulling the wool over your eyes, you are at a serious disadvantage. Politicians, of course, do not want school students studying a subject that tells them when they are being fed a line of nonsense, so they have arranged for logic to be dropped from high school curricula.

There are very few fields of human activity that don't interest some philosophers some of the time. Traditionally, philosophy has concerned itself with The Really Big Questions: the nature and reason for being, the nature of mind, God, ethics and the like. The reason is partly because these are important questions in day to day life, and partly because some people like playing with abstract concepts. Today's abstract concept (the nature of intelligence) becomes tomorrow's hot new technology (artificial intelligence), but, if you need money or popularity, don't think philosophy will do it for you. More likely, somebody else will capitalize on your brilliant philosophical insights and you won't even be offered shares in his company.

Philosophers are very interested in words, because every idea we have must be expressed in words in order to be communicated (there is a very important field called ordinary language philosophy). They want their work to be correct, so they place huge emphasis on the nature of truth, how it can be recognized and so on. This is called **epistemology**. Philosophers expect that if they arrive at what seems to be the truth of a matter, then everybody should fall in line and agree, but this only shows how unworldly they are. Most of the time, most people don't want to be told that what they believe is faulty. They believe it, therefore it can't be wrong. This is true of professors, politicians, police, popes, pimps and pushers alike. It is true of mad men, and it is equally true of philosophers. A philosopher has to be prepared to have his own ideas dissected in public, to have his opponents seize upon his errors and bear them off triumphantly. Any person who says: "I don't think you'll find any errors in my work" is not a philosopher. He may know the language, he may know the jargon and be able to pull his opponent's case to bits with consummate ease, he may even be employed in a philosophy department but, philosophically, he is just another fanatic.

* * *

What should you read if you want to be able to philosophize at your next *soiree*? Essentially, you can read what you like but, if you apply to it the correct, critical attitude, you will find it varies somewhere between mildly interesting but hopelessly out of date all the way down to complete rubbish. Probably the best start is a broad, general history such as Samuel Stumpf's *Socrates to Sartre: a history of philosophy* (about 500 pages), but I'm not sure if it's still in print. Sure, it's high school stuff but it's the sort of thing you can read and put down again. The purpose is to get some idea who was saying what when, so you can see ideas as having lives of their own. This is important: ideas pop up, wave around for a while, and then disappear again for a couple of hundred years. There's nothing new under the sun. Chances are that if you can think of something, then one of those tiresome Greeks or some long-forgotten monk in a monastery in what is now Syria thought of it, too. You need to understand that the smartest people in history are probably not alive today or, if they are, they aren't in a university. Yes, we have amazing technology (like the nifty little smartphone you're holding now) but the ideas aren't new. You like your iPhone? Have a look at the old Dick Tracy comics from 80 years ago. Just keep reminding yourself: there's nothing new under the sun. Even dualism, the idea that I now believe is the correct approach to human mental life, is the oldest of all.

If you have a quiet week, say over Christmas, you could tackle Bertrand Russell's *History of Western Philosophy*. This is very interesting but it presupposes some knowledge of philosophy and can be quite critical in places without letting you know that other people don't see it the same way. At 750 pages, it's getting fairly long. You might like to try one of the *Teach Yourself* books or *Philosophy for Dummies* but I haven't read them and can't say what they are like. You could also stick with the online versions. *Stanford Encyclopedia of Philosophy* will keep you endlessly occupied because, essentially, it's endless. There are plenty of links to other sections of the encyclopedia as well as external links. They don't have a section on history of philosophy but you can look up each section and read the introductions. Mostly, they start easily and lower the reader gently into the heavy duty stuff, as this section from Medieval Philosophy shows:

> "The Main Ingredients of Medieval Philosophy. Here is a recipe for producing medieval philosophy: Combine classical pagan philosophy, mainly Greek but also in its Roman versions, with the new Christian religion. Season with a variety of flavorings from the Jewish and Islamic intellectual heritages. Stir and simmer for 1300 years or more, until done. This recipe produces a potent and volatile brew."

That's the fun bit but if you want to read of a thousand years of human thought in fifteen or so pages, it's a good start and it goes on to dozens of links. What it says is that ideas travel so, if you want to be educated, you need to read. Instead of watching the idiot box or playing online games about warlocks and dragons, try reading Islamic or Indian philosophy. Much more interesting, and more use in the long run. I am told by medical students that nobody reads these days, that the attention span of the average medical student is two minutes for the really interesting stuff. I don't believe it is true of students: they haven't changed that much since I was in school. What is says is that medical schools are pressuring their students to memorize facts at the expense of becoming knowledgeable. Remember this: Education is what's left after you've forgotten everything you were taught (cf. Ambrose Bierce, in his *Devil's Dictionary*: "Education, *n*: That which discloses to the wise and disguises from the foolish their lack of understanding." If you don't know of Bierce, you should).

The *Internet Encyclopedia of Philosophy* doesn't have the same scope as *SEP* but its articles are probably more detailed, so it would not be as helpful to a complete novice. *Wikipedia* has a huge amount of information but the usual problem is finding it. *Wikiversity's* section on philosophy is very patchy so far. Maybe it will get better. It seems that a lot of the books on philosophy on Amazon's Kindle are not meant to be taken seriously (e.g. *The Red Sox and Philosophy*). Apart from the classics, any free books on philosophy are probably worth what you paid for them.

While you're reading background information, don't forget your history of science. John Gribbin's *Science: A history 1543-2001* has enough detail and is suitably reverential. He puts about a hundred of the greats in their context and reminds us how easy we have it today. If you can get a copy of Robert Thompson's *Pelican History of Psychology*, first published in 1968, that does the same thing for all those names who kept appearing, arguing and then disappearing. *Freud and the Post-Freudians*, by JAC

Brown, helps keep tabs on the endlessly schismatic tribes of analysts who had such a profound influence on Western thinking during the twentieth century. Profound, but a total waste of time: Brown shows incisively how psychoanalysis breached all the rules of the philosophy of science.

At the end of this book I have included a glossary of some of the more typical terms you will find in your studies. It is important to know them because you will find that they keep popping up in different guises. All too often, especially in psychiatry, people announce a brilliant new discovery. For a while, everybody mills around in excitement, convinced that this will be the dawn of a new age but, after a while, it slowly fades until, a few years later, a new one bursts on the scene and the old one is forgotten. They are never new. Invariably, they are old ideas tricked out in the latest technobabble and they go nowhere. People need to be able to see through the talk of genes or epigenetics or fMRI scans to find the essential ideas lurking behind the sound bites. History lets us see exactly which intellectual corpse the eager researchers are painting with make-up so they can get their new laboratories or their trips to conferences at the luxury resorts. There aren't that many ideas around, so it doesn't take a lot of effort to be able to recognize them. Standing back from the subject and taking a careful, critical look at it is still the best way to avoid being swept off your feet by nonsense. Especially nonsense peddled by professors.

Chapter 1: Grappling With The Concepts

Until fairly recent times, one of the biggest problems faced by philosophers was the looming shadow of religion. The Church came complete with its own ontology, and churches in general (or synagogues, temples or mosques) are rarely kindly disposed toward competition. Early Christian ontology built on what went before, namely, pagan beliefs, which were intimately related to what we would now call **folk psychology**. That is, every person, no matter how clever or educated or sophisticated, has an immediate and direct knowledge of what it is like to be human: it feels like *something*. A rock, we imagine, doesn't feel like anything, it has no more feeling *of its own* than a bit of finger nail we have pared. But being human is somehow alive and exciting. It brings a knowledge state and a feeling state, so humans can know things and make decisions, and we also have senses and emotions.

All of this adds up to something pretty amazing, which is what the folk psychology version captures: inside each of our heads there is a special something which does all the feeling and sensing and knowing and remembering and deciding that separates us from animals, rocks and dead humans. Most people imagine that the little inner something has the form of a person, so it's usually called a **homunculus**, meaning little man. In this version, your homunculus sits inside your head, checking your visual input on the TV monitors, listening to the loudspeakers from your ears, smelling what you are about to eat and making all the decisions you need to get through you day. The homunculus is the sense of self, the sense of being a me as distinct from your sense of being you which I can't access (also known as the doctrine of privacy). Also, animals have some sort of sense of self (try stealing your dog's favorite toy). We know that animals can sense and can learn simple things but they are pretty limited so we needn't talk more about them.

However, this special something-in-the-head we can all experience directly is special in another respect: nobody has ever seen it. When a person is alive, we are fairly sure his homunculus is busy and on top of things but, when he is dead, he turns into just another lump of meat that needs to be buried fairly quickly. What happened to his homunculus? What is that essential spark, that vital something that we all know is there but nobody has ever seen? Aha, people decided long ago, it must be magic. If the natural world is the world of trees and water and cows and rocks and weather, then the vital spark must be something from beyond the natural world. It must be *super*natural, which means it must have come from the Ultimate Supernatural Source, God. So the soul, God's special innervating spark, must arrive some time before birth and take up residence in the head until, at the instant of death, it decides to abandon ship and head back to the Elysian fields. All cultures have some version or other of this notion as their folk explanation of what activates humans, of what separates us from pigs, trees, rocks and steaks.

You need to understand that we define a homunculus by what it does in the mental life, not by where it came from (such as heaven, the life force in your food etc.) or its shape or particular properties. It is defined by its functional role in the mental economy, not by its provenance or any other properties. The homunculus explains human activity; that is his purpose. Modern versions of homunculi (the plural) claim they do not involve magic but they fill the same role, so they explain nothing that the old soul didn't. It doesn't really matter, as the idea has been around forever.

In the main, religions around the world are pretty intolerant of people messing with their patented message but the ancient Greeks were unusual in that, mostly, they didn't mind people devising their own schemes. Thus, several of the early thinkers raised serious doubts about the idea of a magical soul living inside the head. Socrates wasn't at all clear what went on in the head or where it came from but he was concerned with the concept of a good life. He wandered around asking sticky questions but some people didn't like them. Eventually, when he had annoyed enough people, this was held against him ("impiety and corrupting the young") and he was condemned to death. His pupil, Plato, adhered more closely to the notion of a magical soul living inside the body until it was called to higher duties, so he didn't have the same trouble with the bigwigs. Aristotle doubted this view, arguing instead that the soul and body were essentially related so that the one could not survive without the other. At the moment of death of the body, he said, the soul also dies. His concept is much closer to the modern notion of the mind as a product of the brain than to the old supernatural idea, but it didn't mesh with the Christian idea of an immortal homunculus or soul, so Aristotle's idea fell in a hole for nearly two thousand years.

In the Abrahamic religions (Jewish, Christian and Muslim), the soul was created perfectly by God and implanted in the fetus, probably at the instant of conception. There it remained until the body was no longer suitable for it, and it returned to live forever in harmony with its Creator. That was the original plan; the major religions also accept the idea of the Fall from Grace so that naughty souls went to a bad place where they were handed over to demons to be tormented for eternity as punishment. In this concept, religion has four elements: explanation, inspiration, exhortation and consolation.

In the first place, religion explained the nature of the universe and how humans could do what they did. The explanation came both from the experience of being human (feeling and knowing) and also from watching humans at work and at play, doing things that other animals clearly couldn't. Chief among these were the quintessentially human attributes of speech, nobility (often in short supply), awareness of beauty, art, etc. The bad bits (war and assorted savageries) could be explained either as God's children being naughty because of their Fall from Grace, or as the result of demonic intervention. In a religion, everything has an explanation. In the first place, it explains the folk psychology experience of something vital occupying the inner space behind our eyes. Further, religion inspired people to do better, in their public and private lives, by publicizing the approved local version of the creation and other uplifting moments in religious history. Exhortation was simply the power of religion to insist people follow the rules or suffer the consequences (now and in the future), while consolation was important for people who had not the slightest knowledge of how the universe worked and often had reason to feel they had got a pretty raw deal. If the poor believed that, in the end, all their oppressors would get it in the neck, they were more likely to keep in their place, pay their taxes and not bother the wealthy.

Backed by the full power of the Church, the religious explanation of human experience remained in place for many centuries. People who questioned it rarely went back for a second round. However, in the early part of the seventeenth century, people started to wonder if there might be more to the world than "that's the way God made it." Armed with his new telescope, the philosopher and naturalist, Galileo Galilei (1564-1642), questioned one of the most fundamental beliefs of the Church, the notion that the world is at the centre of the universe. Compounding his sins, he also suggested the heavens weren't perfect. This earned him what was, by their standards, a fairly mild visit to the Inquisition. Suitably chastened, Galileo recanted but, from the Church's point of view, the damage was done, the rot had started.

Soon after, the French polymath, Rene Descartes (1596-1650) began his program of inquiry into the nature of mind. By a process of systematic doubt, he concluded that the existence of the mind or soul is the only certain thing in our lives. As humans, our senses, our memories and our knowledge can be wrong in every respect except this one: that we exist. Simply by asking the question "Do I exist?" we prove incontrovertibly that we do. Even the last man alive would know that he is alive. If he didn't exist, he couldn't ask the question. Everything else in life could be an illusion but the fact that our souls or minds exist cannot be denied: to each individual, it is a real thing. However, Descartes was fully aware that the mind or soul is a special sort of real thing, one which nobody can see. So he arrived at his conclusion, known ever after as "**substance dualism.**" On the one hand, we have the body, which is an ordinary lump of physical substance (it can be localized, seen, cut up and it definitely smells). In this respect, the human body is just a clever physical machine, more or less the same as all other animals have. Descartes was sure that we could give a full account of animals in terms of their physical machinery. However, motivating and controlling our human machine is an entity made of a different sort of non-physical or soul substance. This is the divine spark, put there by God until it is called away. That is, the mind is a real thing (able to move our limbs and tongues) but it is invisible, formless, weightless, colorless, odorless and tasteless. Thus, unlike chimps, the living human is made of two substances, the material substance of the body and the soul-substance of the homunculus.

Immediately, everybody knew there were problems with this idea, namely, that if the soul has no physical properties, how could it interact with the body? How can something that can go through walls pull on strings in the body to move the arms? So we arrive at the classic "mind-body problem" which has kept philosophers in jobs for centuries. In modern terms, we would phrase it this way: Over here, in the physical realm, subject to the laws of thermodynamics and the laws of the space-time continuum, we have an ordinary biological machine of remarkable similarity to that given to chimps (in fact, we have something like 98% of our DNA, if not more, in common with chimps). If the soul is not a physical entity, and is not subject to the same laws, how can it interfere in nature without causing serious and eventually fatal imbalances in the matter-energy equations that govern the natural universe? Clearly, it cannot, which has led people to reject any and every idea that has a dualist element in it. They see this problem, of mind-body interaction, as the defining silliness of any and all dualist models, because dualist models inevitably lead to breaches of the laws of nature.

In modern times, the most vehement rejectionists have included the American philosophers, Daniel Dennett and John Searle. Dennett in particular loathes and detests dualism as prescientific malarkey designed to fool the masses, religious mumbo-jumbo that distracts us from our real task of explaining behavior in natural terms. Science, they say, is about rational explanations of the phenomena of life, so something that can never be seen or found or isolated is forever beyond the reach of science. So, over the years, there have been many attempts to make sense of the human experience within a scientific framework. Before we talk about them, we should look briefly at what is called the Western scientific framework or ontology.

* * *

Starting just before the time of Galileo, in a number of centers around Europe, some strikingly original thinkers decided that the explanation of the universe given by the Church didn't match the facts they observed quite as well as it should. For example, Galileo himself observed sunspots and what we would now call a supernova, meaning the celestial sphere was not fixed and perfect; despite everything the Church had said, he had clear proof that the heavens changed. The Danish astronomer Copernicus amassed huge amounts of evidence to show that the earth could not be the center of the universe, i.e. the universe was heliocentric, not geocentric. William Harvey showed how blood circulated, the first microscopes showed a totally new world waiting to be described, and so on. From this arose the idea that it was no longer good enough to study the classics to find out about the world, the classics were (horror of horrors) more often wrong than right. The new attitude was that facts were all that counted; in the new science, facts always trumped opinions.

So we gained the concept of an empirical science exploring a material (non-supernatural) universe. Now that it seemed God did not interfere daily in the workings of the world, it meant that any conclusion about the nature of the universe could always be overturned by newly observed facts. The entire scientific tradition changed, from the scientist as the person with the best knowledge of the Bible and the classic texts, to the person who could fit the newest facts into the boldest conjectures or theories. In fact, even the name changed: people who looked at the natural world were no longer known as 'natural philosophers' but as scientists (Latin *scientia*, knowledge, fr. Latin *scire*, to know).

For human mental function, the question was simple: is the "vital spark" (which the Church called the soul) a supernatural element or should it be explained in the same, empirical terms as were making such progress in explaining the phenomena of the natural world? With time, the mainstream churches made grudging accommodation with the burgeoning field of natural science, retreating slightly as new discoveries reinforced the notion that the world is just a heap of rocks populated by some clever machines. The next major blow to the religious view came in the mid-nineteenth century, with the publication of Darwin's *Origin of Species*. Actually, the theory of evolution was co-discovered by James Wallace, of whom we hear very little, but that's another story. So, as industry and science transformed our views of the universe, people began looking to the last great holdout of religious belief, the soul. Could this also be explained in the same terms as, say, steam trains and the telegraph? Needless to say, the Church wasn't inclined to admit defeat and fought a rearguard action which is still going on today. Interestingly enough, in Descartes' original writings, in which he had characterized the human body as a non-miraculous, purely physical machine, some people have detected hints that he was heading toward a materialist explanation of the soul but held back because of his (well-founded) fear of the Inquisition. After he saw what had happened to Galileo, Descartes withdrew from publication a book in which he supported the heliocentric view.

It is difficult for us to understand the intense intellectual and emotional shock people experienced following the publication of Darwin's work. We have grown up in a world of constant change, where scientists are given the very greatest respect because they do the intellectual heavy digging that industry then translates into major technological improvements in life style. So, these days, when people try to argue that science will eventually explain the mind, nobody pays much attention: change is the norm, stasis requires explanation. It is the spiritualists who are reeling under the battering of rampant materialist science. But it wasn't always so.

Darwin didn't directly address the question of the soul but, intellectually, there was no doubt where he was heading. In the second half of the nineteenth century, biological science began making huge advances. Louis Pasteur showed that diseases were caused by tiny beasties, not by magic spells, and Rudolph Virchow began the process of putting pathology on a scientific footing. Santiago Ramon y Cajal began to tease apart the ultimate mystery, the brain, and so on. When the remarkable Hermann von Helmholtz developed a rational basis for investigating living organisms, philosophy had to come to terms with the new science. Ideas were on the move, and one of them was the notion that science could reach further and further to explain the ultimate mystery of life, the "vital spark" which the Church still claimed as its own.

In Leipzig, in Germany, a young physician called Wilhelm Wundt was the first to combine Helmholtz's methods with the study of the mind. Wundt (1832-1920) trained as a physician, then worked under Helmholtz for some years. Apparently, he then decided to enter the church, so he studied philosophy. However, he had the novel idea of combining Helmholtz's scientific research methodology with the study of the mind, so he left the church to open a laboratory in Leipzig in 1879. This entered history as the first purely scientific psychology laboratory. Wundt was apparently a very inquisitive person and applied the new methods to anything that caught his fancy. He had a large number of students, many of whom went on to become famous psychologists in their own right. In particular, they studied the physiology and phenomenology of sensation, blurring the borderland with philosophy, which had always had an interest in the nature of experience. So began the generation of the "armchair philosopher" (actually an armchair psychologist), as people sat around in comfortable universities, trying to work out from their direct experience the nature of sensation. From this activity (or inactivity) came the notorious quote: "I'm having an orange after-experience" (if you look at a green light, it leaves an orange after-image). The goal was to understand these matters in materialist terms but, of course, they didn't have the technology. That didn't come for another hundred years (we now explain after-images in terms of depigmentation of the retinal photoreceptors; introspection is useless). However, and despite the interest Wundt was generating, introspection of the mind didn't go away. So, in the last years before World War I, an American psychologist decided a revolution was in order.

John B Watson (1878-1958) was a young and impatient psychologist who realized that all the armchair introspection was going nowhere. The problem, he shouted to anybody who would listen, was that all this talk about a mind or soul or whatever was a load of hooey that was distracting psychology from its real goal, of understanding behavior. There was no point trying to understand the mind because nobody had ever found one. The reason nobody had found one was because it lay outside the area of application of Western materialist science - if it existed at all. There were no rational or empirical methods by which the soul could be investigated, so the goal of a scientific psychology necessarily shifted, from unobservable internal experiences to externally verifiable behavior.

In a polemical paper published in 1913, he proclaimed the "behaviorist revolution," castigating the direction of psychology as a hunt by the blind for the unobservable. A few years later, by which time he was president of the American Psychological Association, he put flesh to his manifesto. He had heard of the work of the Russian physiologist, Ivan Pavlov, but only at third hand. Pavlov had developed a technique of investigating physiological changes which he called 'conditioning.' On next to no solid information, Watson became convinced he could build a general psychology using just Pavlov's technique. Thus the world welcomed **behaviorism**, the first truly anti-spiritualist science of human conduct. Behaviorists set up a program to give a materialist explanation of human behavior, where materialism means "wholly of the natural world." In very short time, behaviorism took off – and so did Watson. A few years later, he was dismissed from his university because of his unbecoming conduct with his secretary, so he went to Madison Avenue, where he made a fortune in advertising.

There are, however, two problems with this story. The first was that the great Pavlov himself didn't believe it was possible to use his laboratory technique to create a general psychology applicable to all human behavior. He didn't even think it was possible to use it to explain all dog behavior. Right to the end of his long and productive life, Pavlov denied that he was a psychologist or that psychologists would ever have any success in their radically materialist program (this is deeply shocking to psychologists, who have always believed Pavlov was one of them). There is no doubt that Pavlov was a thorough-going materialist himself, but he believed that the brain itself would give the clues for a theory of human behavior, and he knew that the science of the 1920s and '30s was a long way from that point.

The second problem with the comfortable psychological myth is that, somewhere along the line, Watson's evangelistic fervor (and he was an overwhelming character) swept a bit wider than perhaps he had intended. His opposition to the spiritual element as magic also came to incorporate the notion of dualism as Aristotle had understood it. Perhaps it was because of the religious way people were raised in those days, or perhaps it was because of the failure of the Wundtian methods of investigation, or maybe just because there was no technological precedent, but Aristotle's idea of a natural or non-magical dualism was dumped in the rubbish bin of history, along with the magical soul. People began looking for any hint of dualism in order to discard it (which, as I will explain later, was a mistake that still echoes today). On both sides of the political spectrum, a harsh, dehumanizing scientific ethos came to dominate the intellectual scene, including the Soviet Union where it quickly identified with radical socialism and thence spread back to Europe.

About fifty years after Pavlov's death, psychologists began to realize the significance of his prediction that they were wasting their time trying to build a science of psychology on his physiological technique of conditioning. To me, it is astounding that it took them so long. One of Pavlov's last papers, written and published in 1937, in the *Psychological Review*, one of the most widely read and influential psychological journals, is entitled: "A physiologist replies to the psychologists." This states in crystal clear terms his reasons why he believed it was futile for academic psychology to use conditioning as the basis for a general psychology. However, this paper was too shocking to the psychologists, so they totally ignored it. It did not enter the history of psychology: indeed, it was as though it had never been written. This is a sublime example of what the philosopher Thomas Kuhn described as simply refusing to see, of which more later.

Notwithstanding the physiologist's dire personal warning, the tradition of Pavlovian or classical conditioning theory continued to dominate academic psychology and daily practice for another half a century. Somewhere in the 1980s, it ran out of steam, and psychology drifted for a while until it popped up with a "new science" called cognitive-behavioral therapy. At the same time, Skinner's Radical Behaviorism in the US was entering its terminal phases. Skinner, as you will recall from your college courses, was the man who put hungry rats in boxes and rewarded them with food when they pressed bars or did other fancy tricks. He was so certain that he had uncovered the secret of predicting and controlling all animal behavior, including the human animal, that, in 1972, he wrote a best-selling book called *Beyond Freedom and Dignity*. This argued that all human behavior, in its entirety, could be understood in terms of the same principles that drove hungry rats to press bars for food. If we really want to control and predict behavior, he said, we have to move beyond thinking in mentalist terms such as freedom and dignity, because they are artifacts. The book sold millions and was required reading for all psychologists and anybody with any sort of scientific or intellectual pretensions. This is remarkable, as it was pure pseudoscience. However, it became Skinner's swansong. Over the next decade or so, people rapidly lost interest in radical behaviorism. By the time Skinner died in 1990, he was very much yesterday's figure. But his work is important in one respect: his was far and away the most thorough-going attempt to write a non-mentalist psychology. He took the idea of dispensing with mentalist concepts further than anybody – and he failed. He didn't fail because of any personal shortcomings but because the project was unattainable. It is not possible to have a non-mentalist account of human behavior.

So cognitive-behavior therapy (or CBT, as the in-crowd know it) took over in American universities just as it had in Europe, quietly overlooking the fact that it is a frankly mentalist account of human behavior. Now this was a bit of a contradiction because psychologists had spent about 75 years loudly telling everybody that all talk of the mind was primitive, non-scientific rubbish, especially when it was psychiatrists talking about egos and ids. Yet here they were, solemnly pronouncing that there is a mind after all, and that it can be investigated and its problems managed by scientific methods, including talking. However, it wasn't just any old talking, especially the silly notion of talking about the Unconscious; they were talking in a controlled manner to make people better by correcting their beliefs and bad habits. So it had to be science – didn't it? No, not in the slightest.

CBT, which is a very limited technology and not a theory at all, is simply recycled mentalism couched in modern-sounding terms. So, these days, psychologists don't talk about mental pain, they say their clients exhibit cognitive dissonance. People don't have hopes or any other vague, mushy notions, they have life-goals (previously ambitions) and behavioral programs (habits), maladaptive responses (bad habits) and negatively-reinforcing nihilistic response patterns (really bad habits). Cognitive behavior therapy is not a theory of mind (because psychologists still don't like talking about minds), it is a tricked up version of the old moral therapy, where caring people point out the errors of the client's ways and remind him always to count to ten before punching the policeman. Of course, they never really got rid of all the other trappings of behaviorism, the relaxation training, the questionnaires, the daily programs and life charts and reinforcement schedules, because it is all designed to conceal one crucial fact: that psychology really doesn't have a theory of the mind. You could say that it has no – *ology* of the *psyche*. A hundred years after Watson boldly threw down the gauntlet and more or less ordered his profession to follow him into the beckoning uplands of a non-mentalist, scientific psychology, they are still poking around in the scrub of a mentalism that isn't. Watson was adamant: there is no way that materialist Western science can come to grips with an entity that nobody can see, locate, measure, weigh or trap in a bottle. In short, he said, the mind is a myth and we have to chuck it out of our science.

So they tried, they tried very hard for three generations but guess what? The mind is back. My gosh, he's a slippery little homunculus but he's not called the mind, of course, he's now known as the cognitive schema or some such term but whatever it is called, he is still doing the same job as a mind. The cognitive schema is still an invisible, colorless, odorless, tasteless, weightless, insubstantial and very slippery thing that nobody can locate in space; that lives inside the head and pulls the strings or presses the buttons that result in observable behavior. It still comes into existence at some stage before birth and vanishes at the instant of death. And it still laughs and slips away when we try to grasp it with the clumsy tongs of materialist science. In real terms, psychology has made no advances since Aristotle.

***

While all this was happening, Freud's psychoanalytic theories were gathering support among psychiatrists. This was especially true in the US after a number of prominent Jewish analysts fled there in the 1930s to escape the Nazis. Like the behaviorists, Freud also put a huge emphasis on the scientific nature of his work but that was the limit of their similarity. Freud's theories were frank mentalism, i.e. they started with the reality of a mind and went from there without ever looking back. Humans were to be seen in mechanistic terms, albeit heavily concealed under the confusion of the ego defenses, but there was no hint of spirituality in his ideas. Everything - morality, enjoyment, religion, duty, creativity, affection - was to be seen in terms of the then bizarre notion of the human mind as a festering, seething cesspool of violent and mostly disgusting drives. However, the problem with his Byzantine theories is that they had no inherent limit. Anybody could, and many did, develop Freud's ideas in any direction they wanted, but there was nothing in the theory itself to say they were wrong. Starting in the late 1950s, and accelerating rapidly thereafter, a reaction developed against psychoanalysis on the basis that its wild, unfettered mentalism was, for want of a better word, plain loopy. To quote the philosopher, Karl Popper, there was no scientific **demarcation criterion** between psychoanalysis and fantasy.

Popper (1902-1994) was born in Austria and began his career in the philosophy of science at an early age. He was very familiar with psychoanalysis from his teenage years (he had known a lot of the original analysts in Vienna before he left for safety in the UK) and immediately used it as an example of pseudo-science. What he wanted was a firm and reliable border between science and **metaphysics**, the classic field in which empiricism doesn't work. Metaphysics is the organized set of beliefs and opinions about the universe and humanity's place in it (applied ontology, you could say), which are not open to empirical confirmation or refutation. If, for example, you firmly believe in the Easter Bunny, then there is no evidence that will convince you the Easter Bunny doesn't exist. In 1922, at the remarkable age of twenty, Popper realized that, intellectually speaking, psychoanalysis was on a par with the Easter Bunny: there was nothing anybody could say or do that would force a committed analyst to admit his theories were wrong. There was so much intellectual leeway and just plain sloppiness built into the theory of psychoanalysis that it could never be proven wrong. Therefore, Popper concluded, psychoanalysis was no different from a religion or a fanatical political system, such as Marxism or his other pet hate, Nazism. Whatever else, psychoanalysis certainly wasn't science.

Fifty years later, psychiatrists began to realize the truth in Popper's opinion. Quietly, they decided they'd better drop psychoanalysis because it was going nowhere and it was becoming downright embarrassing. Influenced by the rabidly antimentalist behaviorist psychologists who were then holding court in universities throughout the US, they decided that what Watson had said many years before was correct: Western science had no means of coming to grips with the slippery notion of a mind. Therefore, they had no option but to discard all talk of the mind in psychiatry. But how could they do this? How could there be a 'science of mental disorder' that didn't have a model of mind? They could have jumped the fence into the world of philosophy and adopted one of their new, materialist models of mind, except nobody in psychiatry in those days had the faintest idea what they were. Fortunately, there was an old idea that had been hanging around for a hundred years or more, the notion that mental disorder just is a disorder of the brain. That is, the mind doesn't enter the equation. Suddenly, the problem disappeared and so psychiatry threw itself into the era of brain chemicals, of fMRI scans, of ECT (electroshock) and drugs, drugs and more drugs. It gave up all talk of human mental disorder as a matter of the mind, replacing it with the notion that mental disorder is not mental at all, just a fancy sort of neurological disease.

This has two interesting corollaries. Firstly, it says that mental problems cannot have psychological causes but the bold new biopsychiatrists didn't worry about that loose end. Their theory could be applied to one and to all: any mental disturbance of any kind was necessarily chemical in nature. Therefore, a man whose business had gone broke, a soldier who had been tortured, a woman whose wastrel husband had abandoned her and the children, or a child whose drunken, brawling parents neglected him, all had a physical disease of the brain and all should be given drugs. Nobody had to talk to them. What a relief: patients' problems could be diagnosed by handing them a questionnaire or, better still, seating them in front of a computer terminal and leaving them to tick the boxes. It meant that psychiatrists, terribly busy people that they are, didn't have to listen to all those tiresome stories and have patients weeping or ranting around their luxurious offices. It meant they could get on with the hugely lucrative business of turning mental patients into neurology patients.

Second, for psychiatrists who held strong religious views (and there are more than you might think), it meant that there was no conflict between mental illness and the notion of a perfect, divinely-anointed soul sent from heaven. It wasn't the soul that was failing, it was the body letting the soul down, i.e. God's bespoke soul remained perfect and without flaw (compare this with Galileo, who found that God's universe wasn't created perfect). Therefore, as is true of surgeons and other real doctors, there was no conflict between their religious beliefs and their daily practice. After the humiliation of their years in the wilderness of psychoanalysis, psychiatrists gratefully moved closer to the rest of the medical fraternity (it would be interesting to know how a devoutly religious psychiatrist felt in the 1950s, having to learn all that irreligious psychoanalytic stuff, but there probably aren't many left from that era).

* * *

Unfortunately, there is a catch to this comfortable story. It has to be understood that the notion that mental disorder is just brain disorder is not an idea floating free in intellectual space. It is not a stand-alone idea that owes nothing to other ideas. You cannot say: "Two plus two equals four, salt is NaCl and by the way, mental disorder is just brain disorder." People are entitled to object; they are entitled to ask: "Fine, but what's your justification for making that claim?" What they mean by that is something like: "What are the nested beliefs on which that claim depends for its intellectual authority? State them explicitly so that I can see if there are any faults in your reasoning." This points to another feature of Western science, that nothing is accepted on authority. Religion is accepted on authority, political power is accepted on authority (if you know what's good for you), the cricket umpire's decision is accepted on authority, but any nuisance is entitled to ask of any scientist making any claim: "What's your warrant? Put up your evidence or shut up."

The corollary to this is that all scientific claims have to be made in public and anybody and everybody can have a go at duplicating them, or disproving them. In the main, a scientific claim carries no weight until somebody else has duplicated it, preferably by a different method. There is no such thing as an unsubstantiated scientific claim. But the claim "mental disorder is just brain disorder" is an unsubstantiated scientific claim. It is a *metaphysical* claim, meaning a claim which cannot be decided by empirical evidence. However, the way orthodox psychiatrists use it, it is a metaphysical claim masquerading as a scientific or empirical claim. Once again, it is the type of claim for which Popper derided the Freudians: there is no evidence that could convince a committed biopsychiatrist that he is wrong (again, you see there's nothing new under the sun). Now, you have to put aside any thoughts that this claim may be very reasonable, or that it makes sense or it's very tidy, or that it does the major world religions a favor. All that counts in science is this: is there any conceivable evidence that could prove that claim one way or the other? If there is not, then it isn't a scientific claim. It is a metaphysical claim and anybody who acts as though it is a proven truth, who acts as though it is a scientific fact, is embracing it for **ideological** reasons. An ideologue is a person who holds strong metaphysical views and refuses to consider they may be wrong. We tend to reserve the term for people who hold very strong, unwavering political views but it also means a fanatical religious believer. Ideologues are not nice people. At best, they are intolerant and domineering but, at their worst, they are homicidal, if not genocidal. There is no room in science for ideologues. Are biological psychiatrists ideologues?

To answer that, we will need to make an excursion through some ideas about the mind. First, we can define science: **Science** is a rational, empirical endeavor directed at understanding the matter-energy relationships throughout the universe. It is rational because it is rule-governed, and the rules are freely available to anybody. The rules are determined in advance: if you want to investigate the life at the bottom of your fish pond, there are certain things you can do and certain things you can't do. For example, you have to follow particular procedures in a set order and you have to keep detailed records that must be published for somebody else to duplicate your work. There is no secrecy in science: all scientific information has to be shared. That applies even in secret military laboratories, because somebody else on the project will have to inspect the process and criticize it (this is partly why German science, then the world's best, ground to a halt under the Nazis: nobody was allowed to criticize something Hitler liked).

Science is empirical, meaning it is about facts. There are no opinions about those facts that cannot be overturned by further evidence. This means that the scientific project never ends. Somebody can always find a new fact somewhere, and the race is on again. It is an endeavor because it has no central plan and no defined goal: nobody knows where science will be in ten years' time. Huge numbers of people are involved, most of them pursuing some childhood dream despite the drudgery, but there isn't a predetermined master plan. Somebody gets an idea, everybody rushes after it, the main idea goes nowhere but, in an obscure laboratory far away, some bright young thing realizes a critical point that everybody else has overlooked, and a new rush develops. Science does not go in straight lines. The impression of a grand highway leading from ignorance to light is just an impression (put about, in the main, by ideologues).

Science is directed at understanding the matter-energy relationships throughout the universe. That is, it is locked into understanding the natural, material universe. There is a gigantic firewall between science and any supernatural ideas. Science deals with facts using objective tools; anything that cannot be grasped by those tools lies outside the scientific arena. Hence the historical difficulty of Western science in dealing with the mind: there are no independently verifiable, objective facts of the mind. By definition, the mind is subjective, which places it neatly but firmly on the other side of that firewall. There, it can amuse the religious, the ideologues and philosophers while the scientists get on with finding a cure for the cancers that kill the religious, the ideologues and philosophers, just as effectively as they kill nice people.

There is one problem with this neat way of cutting the universe into rational and irrational bits: not everything that is rational can be investigated under a microscope. For example, 2+2=4 is perfectly rational but it cannot be investigated using the materialist scientific methodology. You think it can? OK, try putting these in a centrifuge:

"Acceleration of the gross annualized per capita national deficit on a log scale."

"Your action is insulting to our national heritage and any repetitions will be deemed acts of war."

It doesn't work, believe it. There cannot be a non-mentalist explanation of human behavior. So the definition of science has to be widened, thus: Materialist science investigates the matter-energy relationships throughout the universe *and the informational states controlling them*. Now we have thrown the net over computers and other rational machines, the only question is whether it is good enough to deem the human mind a "rational machine." Sometimes, it seems pretty irrational.

So, when biological psychiatrists claim that "mental disorder is just brain disorder," are they making a scientific claim or are they just being ideologues? Let's dive back into history again.

* * *

By the second half of the nineteenth century, the whole intellectual world was in ferment. Politically, the reverberations of the French and American revolutions were still rolling around the world. In Europe, radical socialism was a rising force, tending to combine with anarchic republicanism and provoking vicious reactions from (you guessed it) reactionaries. In science, the rapidly developing fields of electricity and chemistry were transforming the laboratory and industry, while biology was still reeling from Darwin's explosive work. Art, finance, exploration: the world was booming. In philosophy, revolution was threatening. People were no longer so intimidated by the church and were prepared to push the boundaries as far as they could. A split, which is still with us, began to develop between the world of Continental philosophy and the Anglo-American schools. Under the influence of the German Georg Hegel, European philosophy turned to the idea that the world could be understood just by exploration of one's inner experience. From this, after about 150 years and mountains of print, arose what is now called the Continental or phenomenological school of philosophy. This is diametrically opposed to the Anglo-American tradition which is concerned with analysis. It is my opinion that phenomenology is one of the outstandingly successful con jobs in intellectual history. I have outlined my case in Chapters 4 and 5 of my book, *Humanizing Psychiatrists* (published in 2010), so, with relief, we can cut the Continent loose and let it drift noisily over the horizon. Unfortunately, we are a bit late: the cancer of phenomenology has well and truly metastasized to the rational world.

This side of the water, a new tradition developed, very much part of the Enlightenment tradition of rule-governed, objective intellectual inquiry. When science began to split from philosophy, some time in the seventeenth century, the rump didn't wither and die. Instead, it went from strength to strength, developing in new and completely unexpected directions. Essentially, Anglo-American philosophy consists of rigorous analysis of a wide range of topics, the common feature being an objective, abstract and rule-governed inquiry into the nature and meaning of activities and entities. For example, there is a very broad field concerned with meta-analysis of language. What is language? How do we communicate? How is meaning encoded in sounds or in scrawls on pages? How does language relate to the brain, to society, to history and to machines? It's a huge and growing field which has direct entry to such fields as semantics, semiotics, computers and IT, artificial intelligence, and so on. Very interesting, but also fiendishly difficult.

Another field is the philosophy of science, which is about what can be studied in science, how it should be studied, how science progresses and, of course, the ethics of science. We will come back to this in a separate chapter. Logic, of course, goes from strength to strength, partly because of its central role in IT. The study of knowledge and understanding has become a specialty in its own right: **epistemology.** *The Cambridge Dictionary of Philosophy* defines it as "…the study of knowledge and its justification, specifically a) the defining features, b) the substantive conditions, and c) the limits of knowledge and justification." What can we know, how do we know, what can we believe, what is the nature of belief? All of these are questions for epistemologists, but all philosophers have to be familiar with them. Metaphysics is still with us, as are ethics and many new, applied fields: the philosophy of education, of the environment, of war (still), of government, of law and so on. All of these fascinating fields share the English-speaking tradition of rule-governed, objective intellectual inquiry (there are still continental schools of rational inquiry, but they struggle to be heard over the din of phenomenology).

Still, the central preoccupation, if not fixation, of philosophy is the human being. What is the nature of the controlling element in human affairs? How is it formed, where does it come from, how does it relate to the body, and so on. These questions will be considered (note I didn't say 'answered') in the next chapter.

Chapter 2: Grappling With A Single Mind

In talking about the concept of mind, it is probably easiest to start with the simplest version, the one our grandmothers acquired early in their lives. This is what has been termed the 'folk psychology' version of the mind (the name comes from Wilhelm Wundt, who produced twenty thick books about it). As mentioned in the previous chapter, the notion is of a 'little man' (or 'little woman') residing in the head and doing everything that humans do that we can't already understand as something ducks and dogs do. So, language, creativity, art, chivalry and so on have to be explained in terms other than of simple mechanisms bumping and clicking in the dark. But, the inquisitive child will invariably ask, where does the little man come from? "God," says grannie in a tone that says "and that is the end of your questions, run off and play." Perhaps the child goes to the priest and says: "Where does the little man come from?" "God," replies the priest, "and bless you, my son, but I have a sermon to prepare." So the child goes along the road and wonders: If humans have little men inside them, perhaps animals do, too. What about trees? Everybody knows trees are very noble things, they should have one, too. And so this train of thought leads directly to two ancient ideas, **animism** and **panpsychism**.

Animism is generally accepted as the primal religion. It simply says that everything has spirits inside it, many of which mischievous, and often they have to be placated. If you go out at night, especially on a dark and stormy Friday 13th, you will be in danger because that is the night the spirits come out and party. On a spring morning, if you go to a hidden glen, and sneak up quietly, you may find the spirits out frolicking in the morning sunlight, perhaps even bathing and combing their silken locks but beware. It is forbidden for humans to see the spirits and woodland nymphs and they may send a demon after you, perhaps to capture you and taunt you for eternity, or simply to make your life a misery, breaking your hoe or letting your goat snap its rope and wander off. Traditional Australian Aboriginal culture was animistic, for example, they believed that women became pregnant at about 18wks, at the time of quickening, i.e. the first fetal movements were the spirit entering them as an infant. This was part of their totemic system which was so complicated that nobody else understood it.

Animists tend to be fairly respectful of the spirits they believe can benefit them or hurt them, but don't feel the same about the rest of life. Taken to its limit, they would have to accept that every bacterium has a spirit and should be treated carefully, which makes eating your yoghurt or the yeast in your bread or beer a bit difficult. Animism is still widespread. In most cultures, the ancient religions are not lost when a new religion arrives, they are simply taken over. For example, the so-called Easter Bunny was a Celtic fertility rite (rabbits being especially fertile little creatures), and the Christmas tree was a sign of rebirth in mid-winter. A lot of Thai culture is pre-Buddhist, for example, the little spirit houses that people place in their gardens. In Java, Islam arrived late, after the Hindus and the Buddhists, giving a unique fusion of animistic beliefs (especially fortune telling), Hindu sagas (the Ramayana) and a mild-mannered Islam. The late President Suharto always consulted his soothsayer before any major decisions, and public events often have to fit in with the spiritual calendar. This, of course, has nothing to do with modern philosophy but it has a lot to do with people and culture.

Panpsychism is only one step removed from animism. It says that the human mind is assembled from little bits of mentality that inhere in all matter. When enough bits come together, preferably in the right pattern, then a little mental man will be assembled. So panpsychists believe that everything is sentient, and therefore entitled to some protection, except that humans have to get enough of their bits to stay alive, and they get it through their diet. Mosquitoes, for example, can be shooed away but they should not be killed. However, when something dies, it decomposes into its constituent atoms, and each atom has its own bit of sentience and so the cycle starts all over again. This is not so far removed from the original Buddhist teachings so you see that ideas have a habit of popping up in different guises at different times and in different cultures.

The problem with panpsychism is that it doesn't actually explain mentality, it just says it has always been and is part of the natural cycle of life. It leads to difficulties, such as believing that rocks should be treated with respect because they have structure and organization, and therefore have spirits of their own, whereas bad humans can be chopped up and fed to the fish because it's good for the fish. The philosopher, David Chalmers, briefly invoked panpsychism in his account of dualist models of mind but it wasn't meant to be taken seriously, only showing that panpsychism could account for emergence: "There seems to be no knockdown arguments against the view," he said, "and there are various positive reasons why one might embrace it." That may be logically true but, in a materialist science, we need not take it seriously because it cannot be proven. If we can't detect any movement in them, there is no way of knowing whether rocks have consciousness. Therefore, panpsychism is inseparable from religion, i.e. it is a matter of metaphysics but not of science, so we can move along.

You can see, then, that the standard Christian notion of the supernatural soul is a logical development of these ideas. Simply, all the soul-stuff in the universe has been harvested and placed in a heavenly silo, where God uses it to fashion new souls for all the dear little children who are being bred by their wanton parents. When the new body is ready, or maybe at the moment of conception, the soul is dispatched to its new abode. There it resides for the next few decades until it decides that arthritis isn't such a great thing and is relieved when a heart attack (possibly from the anti-arthritis drugs) ends its sentence and lets it wing its way aloft again. Note that these are all dualist ideas, i.e.

they regard soul-stuff and material-stuff as two distinct orders of being which have to interact by some unstated means. This is the rub: Western science is materialist, it uses the laws and principles of the material universe to investigate itself but it cannot use those laws to investigate something that doesn't obey them. How could you trap a soul in a glass beaker if it can simply glide through the walls? "OK, soul, I'm just going to take your temperature with this rectal thermometer… Hey, where did you go? Come back, that's not fair."

So, over the centuries, there has been a steady drift of opinion among scientists that "something must be done" about the spirit. We have already seen one of their efforts - behaviorism, which ruled the spirit out of order and tried to assemble a science of all human conduct (behavior) without letting any spiritual or dualist elements in their chain of explanation. It didn't work, and if you would like to see some of the problems they ran into, you could do worse than read Noam Chomsky's devastating critiques of Skinner's work, especially of his books *Verbal Behavior* and *Beyond Freedom and Dignity* (an online reference is at the end of this book). Chomsky's crit of *Verbal Behavior* was printed in 1959 and, from then on, Skinner's days were numbered. It is brilliant and devastating, perhaps second only to Peter Medawar's stunning critique of the French Jesuit and crank, Teilhard de Chardin. The process accelerated in 1971 when his critique of *Beyond Freedom and Dignity* left Skinner's scientific reputation in tatters. You may ask, How could anybody as smart as Skinner be so catastrophically wrong? I think the answer is that this is a very good example of what happens when scientists spend all their time working and talking with people who agree with them. Skinner must have circulated his books in his department before they were published. They were all committed behaviorists, so they wouldn't have seen the faults, or perhaps it was just a case of the emperor's new clothes.

It is an interesting comment on scientists that, throughout the time that generations of psychologists were spending millions attempting to build their "brave new non-mentalist world," there was practically no serious philosopher in the world who thought they could do it. The acerbic Alfred Ayer, one of the pre-eminent English philosophers of the first half of the century, said that claiming to be a behaviorist was akin to claiming to be anesthetized from the neck up. Popper thought behaviorists were a joke, and often used Skinner as an example of pseudo-science. He was of the view that conditioning didn't actually exist, and therefore did not believe that it could be used as the basis of a general psychology. In his *History of Western Philosophy*, Bertrand Russell hardly mentioned psychologists or behaviorism. He believed Pavlov's physiological principle of the conditioned reflex could not be generalized to account for mental life: "I do not wish to exaggerate the scope of the conditioned reflex," he said, exactly at the time psychologists were desperately trying to exaggerate it. Continental philosophers, of course, didn't take the slightest notice of behaviorists (not that that is a recommendation). Back here in the dull world of science, the assembled physicists and pathologists and mathematicians and geologists couldn't have cared less what the psychologists were doing, let alone the philosophers. They could use their minds to pursue their research but didn't need to know how minds worked. It is the same as a farmer, who uses his back and his arms and his eyes to plough his fields but doesn't have a clue how backs, arms or eyes work. As long as they work, he doesn't need to.

This is an important view of science. If you learn only about science in textbooks written by scientists, or from lectures given by scientists, or seminars organized by scientists to encourage you to study science, or from the many articles, TV shows, websites etc. devised and posted by scientists to convince the world they need more money, then you might, just might, get the idea that science is a very noble calling, that scientists are valiantly dispelling the forces of darkness by shining the light of their brave minds through the fog of ignorance, something like that. It isn't true, of course. Scientists are very narrow-minded, inward-looking and just as prone to the human foibles and weaknesses as any other group. Probably more so, because their personal involvement in their research is enormous. For a millionaire fighting to defend his pile, it's only money and there's more where that lot came from. However, for a scientist, all is ego; winning the argument is all, and nothing else matters. That's why it has been said that academic battles are the most vicious, because all that hangs on them is academic egos.

The scientific endeavor is tightly focused in on itself. Instead of seeing Science Triumphant as a steadfast knight in shining armor, forging his way ahead into the shrinking fields of night, it is better to see the field of science as a small field surrounded by a high fence, in which large numbers of people huddle jealously over their bit of turf, trying to see what is going on the next group while concealing their plot, and totally ignorant of what is happening up there on the hills surrounding their little cantonment. By degrees, this whole, vast edifice actually does something. It builds a structure; sure, bits fall off and there are tantrums and cries of sabotage but, with the passage of time and large sums of money, it advances. I think it was ego that prevented psychologists seeing that their behaviorist project was doomed from the beginning. Ego, and more than a little ignorance.

* * *

While the behaviorist experiment was playing itself out, what were the philosophers doing? In fact, they were very busy. In the US, there was an essentially homegrown movement called **pragmatism** which tried to characterize the meaning of a statement in terms of its utility. The first exponent of this eminently practical philosophy was the remarkable Charles S Peirce (pronounced Purse), who was followed by William James (brother of Henry and Alice, no relation to Jesse) and John Dewey. As its name suggests, pragmatism was directed at finding relatively non-contentious ways of settling disputes over meaning and other complex epistemological questions.

In Britain, at about the same time, the philosophical world was astounded by the scholarship of Russell and Whitehead's monumental *Principia Mathematica* and, between the wars, by the searing brilliance of the decidedly unstable Ludwig Wittgenstein. In 1949, another bombshell landed, Gilbert Ryle's *The Concept of Mind*. This was a rather unusual book in that it set out to dispel what he called the myth of Cartesian dualism by means of ordinary language philosophy. Today, and despite its wealth of prosaic examples, it is not an easy book to read, partly because it isn't always clear what he is trying to disprove: we have changed, too. He mounts a sustained attack on the notion of the "ghost in the machine," the classic dualist understanding of Descartes' position, but is not at all clear on what should take its place. He does not characterize himself as behaviorist, yet it would be fair to say that a lot of his argument is monist in nature, i.e. he is claiming that, in some vital sense, mind and body are one and the same thing, without specifying the nature of the relationship. In the decades following this book, and, to some extent, because of it, philosophy changed quite dramatically, but not always in directions that Ryle would have appreciated.

By the 1950s, the Cartesian model of substance dualism was in full retreat. People had very largely given up trying to make sense of it because nobody had any suggestion as to how the different substances could interact. The emphasis shifted to **monism**, i.e. accounting for the phenomena of mind and body within the context of the material universe (there is an alternative form of monism, that everything is mental, but it is essentially a religious viewpoint so we won't pursue it). There were many variants of monism, and the differences sometimes seemed less real to observers than to the squabbling academics guarding their territories. What follows is essentially a list of – isms, most of which are now only of historical interest but it is important to know of them so they can be recognized each time they are recycled after yet another bout of cosmetic surgery. They were all designed to get over the insuperable hurdle of dualist interaction (and yes, I know you can't get over an insuperable hurdle, that's what insuperable means, but the point is to go around it, not over it).

Perhaps the simplest form of monism is **epiphenomenalism**, which says, yes, there are two realms, but only one matters. The phenomena of mind are, in fact, epiphenomena of the real action in the brain, which takes place at the level of neurons and chemicals. Mental events do occur but they are harmless and ineffective shadows of what is going on at the chemical level, so we don't have to explain them. They are no more causative of behavior than the steam over a factory causes the action on the factory floor. Noise, for example, is an epiphenomenon of a door slamming, as it is for an electric guitar, even though for the musical instrument, it is the rationale. We strike a piano's keys to produce an epiphenomenon, just as the monitor display on the computer I am using is an epiphenomenon: I can switch it off if I like and continue to type just as effectively (especially if the Spellcheck is left on). There is a lot to be said for this approach, e.g. we don't actually think about most of what we do, but they are still our actions, effective, goal-directed or any other test you care to apply. Unfortunately, epiphenomenalism doesn't say anything about what is happening at the effective level of mind. If we say what the mind is not, we have not said anything interesting about what the mind is. It says only that, at the effective or functional level of what we call mind, mind and body are of one and the same order of being. Mental events, such as the experience of seeing red or tasting sour, are of no causal significance and don't need to be explained.

"Who cares about the color red," an epiphenomenalist would say, "the real action is neuronal."

"OK," you reply, "so what about a little friendly torture, then? Is pain an epiphenomenon or does pain *cause* you to pull away?"

"All will be explained at the neuronal level," your opponent snorts. "Pulling away from a noxious stimulus is only a neuronal event, even worms do it." Suddenly, he is falling into the trap, not of explaining something, but of *explaining it away*. There is a big difference.

The problem for the epiphenomenalist is to show how mental actions can be explained in non-mentalist terms, which is the old problem the behaviorists couldn't overcome. In a sense, he could say he doesn't need to explain mentalist things such as wanting a drink, because dogs also seem to want a drink, and we don't demand a mentalist explanation for them. Well, that may be just speciesism, but I can also think of mental events that dogs can't do (writing a criticism of the notion of a just war, for example, or budgeting for next week's holiday). I might be prepared to give the epiphenomenalist some credence if and only if he could indicate some path by which mental events could have a neuronal explanation. However, that probably won't happen because the world has moved on. Nobody takes epiphenomenalism seriously these days.

Mind-brain identity theory states that, as a matter of fact, mind and brain are one and the same thing. This is not intuitive, because of the old objections: I can weigh a brain but I can't weigh a mind. Brains can be localized to one spot in the head while minds evade every attempt to find a spot for them. But it solves one problem: if mind and body are of the same order of being, there is no difficulty about mental events hopping over into the brain to kick start it each morning. Again, it says nothing about the nature of the brain's activity in controlling the hand that is designing the sculpture or writing the poem but that is left to the future, which becomes an example of what is called **promissory materialism.** This says: Don't worry, the scientists will ride to the rescue. One day, they will explain the mind and all those loose ends in terms of neuronal activity and everybody will be happy.

This isn't as dippy as it sounds. There have been many examples of science clearing up major problems, such as earthquakes, disease, even babies, but they were problems of a fairly particular kind. As problems, they fell squarely within the natural or material realm, so Western materialist science had no real difficulty dealing with them. However, the first question a promissory materialist would have to answer is whether mental matters rightly belong to the class of questions that materialist science can be expected to solve. Most people would say that, fairly clearly, the mind is *not* in that realm. That is the issue. It's not good enough to say, "Well, we scientists gave you supersonic jets and iPhones, so we can sort out the problem of sonnets in the same way, just give us enough time (and money) and you'll see." They might be leading us on another chase like the search for the philosopher's stone or the fountain of youth or the perpetual motion machine. Science does not claim to be able to solve all problems, only the problems for which it was designed. It doesn't solve metaphysical questions or questions of values or anything distinctively human. It is very important to be on the alert for examples of promissory materialism. They can be very subtle and are enormously popular with scientists (who get new laboratories and big expensive toys to play with) and, ominously, politicians, who can shift the problem to the over-eager scientists and then blame them when it doesn't work out. Biological psychiatry is currently the best example of a field which may yet turn out to be just promissory materialism on the rampage.

Another version of this is **eliminative materialism,** which says that what seem to be two incommensurable orders of being will turn out to be one, after all. Given sufficient scientific progress, the notion of a mind will be eliminated. The classic example is the theory of phlogiston, the hidden "essence" which was released when an object burned. With a better theory, i.e. chemical combustion leading to release of energy, science eliminated the notion of phlogiston. Another is the old idea of the ether, a sort of cosmic fluid that was thought to be necessary if waves (such as light and other forms of EM radiation) could travel through space. In a classic demonstration called the Michelson-Morley experiment, it was shown that the speed of light was the same in any direction and at any time of the year. Because of the Doppler effect, this would not be possible if the ether were moving (which it would be relative to us because of the earth's orbit around the sun). This soon led to a major crisis in classic physics, from which arose Einstein's concept of relativity and the world has never been the same. Again, scientific progress eliminated a false theory.

People use these examples to "prove" that mental life is a misconception of the order of phlogiston or the ether but they are making a mistake. The reason it doesn't make sense is this: phlogiston and the ether were attempts at explanations of observations. They were themselves invisible theoretical constructs. I am not using my mental experiences to explain anything. I want somebody to explain my mental life itself, to explain my sense of being something able to cause my hands to type these words or scratch my head. My mentality is a brute fact of my life, and that fact is what needs explaining. You cannot eliminate my mental life by scientific progress. There is, as Descartes showed, no evidence you can put before me that will convince me I don't exist. That's what I want explained, that sense of being something able to act on the real world.

Returning to mind-brain identity theory (MBIT), it didn't go far because it was quickly apparent that minds and brains are not, in fact, identical: minds have properties that brains don't have, and vice versa. For example, minds have the color green but brains don't. Obviously, there is more to their relationship than simple identity. Aha, said its proponents, but have you forgotten the example of the morning star? The morning star and the evening star are, in fact, one and the same thing: the planet Venus. Fine, but that shifts the argument somewhat. What we now have is an example of **neutral monism,** the idea that neither mind nor brain are what they appear to be as they are both examples of a third entity which we haven't yet sorted out. But watch this space, neutral monists say, because scientists will soon fill it, i.e. promissory materialism lifts its beguiling head again.

Isn't this fun? We have a problem. Somebody suggests a solution, then everybody jumps on it and tears it to bits. Meantime, the author has a great time signing his books at conferences in exotic resorts, so everybody wins. But that's how any intellectual endeavor progresses. Without criticism, there is no progress.

There were several other attempts at monist theories during the 1950s and 60s but I have to admit I can't see the difference between them and one or other of the types described above. It becomes an exercise in splitting hairs (which philosophers love) but it goes nowhere, so perhaps it's time to move on to the two Really Big Cheeses in the modern theory of mind, reductionism and functionalism.

Reductionism is what you might expect: the notion that something big can be fully explained by reducing it to its bits and seeing how they fit together. There are two main sorts of reductionism, **ontological reductionism** and **behavioral reductionism**, but they really aren't that different. Ontological reductionism states that the properties of a higher order entity can be fully explained in terms of the properties of its lower order constituents. Behavioral reductionism states that the behavior of a higher order entity can be fully explained in terms of the behaviors of its lower order constituents. You might object that the behavior or an entity just is one of its properties, and I wouldn't disagree, but some people have seen a difference. But let's deal with ontological reductionism, because that is probably the most successful single intellectual endeavor in human history. It is usually known just as reductionism, and it is the essential basis of practically the whole of modern science and technology.

If you want to know what a rock is, you have a look and make a detailed list of all the crystal types you can see. Then you break each crystal down, and down, and down until you get to something that can't be broken down further. All the properties of the rock, its size, weight, density, conductivity, coefficient of expansion and so on, are the cumulative properties of those final elements, namely, its atomic elements. Why atomic? Because that's what the word means: *a-*, Gk. not, and *–tomic*, Gk. can be broken. *Atomic,* cannot be broken, an adjective, from which the English noun is *atom*, except we now know that atoms are composed of little subatomic particles. So the properties of any uniform entity just are the composite properties of its final elements, and the properties of its elements are determined by the properties of its sub-atomic particles. The properties of a non-uniform entity, such as a plant or a hand drill or a kidney, are the properties of its constituent parts. By taking the machine apart (plants and kidneys are just biological machines), we can see how each bit fits together so that matter and energy can travel through the system to produce its output. That is the essence of any material machine: it manipulates physical inputs, meaning chemicals and energy, according to predetermined pathways, to achieve an output that would be vanishingly unlikely if that machine did not exist. In doing so, it obeys the laws of physics to a T; there can be no breach of any of these laws, especially thermodynamics.

For example, a hand drill allows neat holes to appear in a piece of wood. If we were prepared to wait long enough, the hole might appear itself (say by very upright wood worms, or an unusual form of wood rot) but, given what we know about the nature of the world, that is exceedingly unlikely. However, given the form and structure of a hand drill, and given a particular energy input, then the drill bit will turn and the wood will be drilled. Thermodynamically, it is not impossible for the holes to appear spontaneously, but don't count on it. Thus, a machine does not do anything magic, it simply manipulates the laws of thermodynamics to achieve an otherwise exceedingly unlikely goal. Enzymes do this as well. An enzyme does not force an impossible chemical reaction, it simply increases the likelihood of an unlikely reaction by many orders of magnitude. Some biochemical reactions are catalyzed at rates many hundreds of millions of times beyond their unassisted or natural rates, but there is no breach of the laws of thermodynamics as the catalyzed reaction consumes energy and increases entropy.

So reductionism is a very powerful form of explanation, the most powerful we know. It is so powerful and so pervasive that it is almost our automatic response: if there's a problem, have a look inside. Your car's stopped? Let's have a look inside. The stove doesn't work? Let's have a look inside. You don't feel well? Let's have a look inside. In brief, reductionism is the ultimate form of explanation in the material world, just because everything in the material world is composed of smaller elements. Given the laws of the natural world, and the physical structure, we can explain anything. Anything? Well, what about explaining the pain in my finger.

"Ah," says the committed reductionist, "it's all a matter of nerves and neuro-transmitters and the brain. It all reduces to neuronal activity."

"Now hold on a moment," you reply. "You said everything can be explained in terms of its constituents. The weight of a rock is the weight of its atoms. The output of carbohydrates by a chloroplast is the result of its input of carbon, oxygen, water and sunlight. So how does a neuron in my brain cause a sense of pain? Are you suggesting all the neurons have a little bit of pain and it all adds up to a big pain for me? At the same time, is my sense of self the additive result of a lot of little senses of selves in my neurons? And why stop at neurons? They have subcellular organelles, and in turn, they are composed of complex molecules, and they of atoms. Where does your reductionism stop?"

You won't get an answer. The committed reductionist accepts that what works for *Aplysia* (sea slugs) will work for humans. Anyway, we're not sure that it works for *Aplysia*; maybe they have a very rudimentary sense of pain if they get an electric shock.

The question is: how can we reduce mental properties to physical elements? Isn't there a contradiction there? We are trying to give an account of two incommensurable orders of being, and simply announcing that what works for rocks will work for the highest reaches of the human experience is not convincing in the slightest. In fact, it sounds awfully like the way the teachers used to talk in Sunday School: This is the truth, and you'd better believe it. Well, as I said above, my view is: Without criticism, there is no progress.

As always, the burden of proof of reductionism rests with those who make the claim. The null hypothesis is that reductionism does not explain the human experience. Anybody who claims that it does is assuming a heavy burden of proof, so let's have a look at what they are claiming, and the proof they are providing. Where can we start? I know, let's start with a well-known neurophysiologist, coincidentally, the one who got a Nobel Prize for his work on *Aplysia*. Eric Kandel is one of the most senior professors at Columbia Medical College in New York. In his most recent books, including his autobiography (*In Search of Memory: the emergence of a new science of mind*, 2006) and a collection of his papers (*Psychiatry, Psychoanalysis and the New Biology of Mind*, 2005), he explicitly states that biological reductionism will answer the problems of mind and of psychiatry. The first lines in his autobiography spell this precisely: "Understanding the human mind in biological terms has emerged as the central challenge for science in the twenty-first century. We want to understand the biological nature of perception, learning, memory, thought, consciousness, and the limits of free will." If you would like to read more details of his claim, they are set out at length in Chap. 1 of my second book, *Humanizing Psychiatry* (2009).

Of course, Kandel isn't the only person making this claim; psychiatrists have been saying the same thing ever since they gave up on psychoanalysis. In mainstream psychiatry, it is now accepted without question that biology will deliver the goodies. It is not quite a matter of promissory materialism, it is more a case of "We have the model, all we need is a bit of time (and money) and we will be able to answer any question about the human mind. Any question." OK, well here's one. Tell me how, without some additional information, you would be able to look at a brain and decided its recent user spoke Hindi with a Punjabi accent, or Swahili with a Kenyan accent? If you doubt this, go to www.ted.com and search for Gero Miesenboeck. In the first couple of minutes, this elegant lecture shows the sheer impossibility of being able to look at a brain and work out what it is doing just from the evidence of your eyes alone.

In fact, it is not just a matter of practical impossibility, it is a logical impossibility. Mind-brain reductionism is impossible in any conceivable world, including Eric Kandel's laboratory in New York. It is impossible because, in order to "read off" the informational content of the brain (or its neurons, or its subneuronal elements, its molecules or atoms, it makes no difference), you need to know the codes in which the information is stored. And the brain cannot tell you that. It doesn't know its codes, any more than the heart "knows" how it contracts. Not even the owner of the brain could tell you, because he has no access to his brain (in truth, not one of us even knows he has a brain. I've seen a shadow of mine on a CT scan but that proves nothing, maybe the radiologist was just trying to reassure me).

"Aha," your committed biological reductionist crows, "you're wrong. We could open the skull, put in the probes and then ask the person what he was thinking. After a few zillion trials, we would learn his codes."

Maybe. Maybe you would learn the codes used by the brain's 100 billion neurons, but I doubt it, and not just because there's a lot of them (using about 100 neuro-transmitters for a start, and that's just the latest count). But let's say you did learn the code the brain was using today, what about tomorrow? Today, the password is *Red Dog*; tomorrow, it's *Blue Cat*. It still opens the door. That is, the codes can change, infinitely. While we're at it, let's talk about mathematics. How can a finite machine called the brain generate an infinite output? Same goes for language; the finite brain can generate an infinite number of sentences in an infinite number of languages. An infinite output cannot be mapped back onto a finite substrate (I saw yesterday that the English language now has just over a million words. That means the chances of this sentence arising spontaneously are 10^{-60}. Somehow, I think ordinary language would overload even the best probes). Maybe you could learn my codes, but how would anybody know that every human uses the same codes? Perhaps we all learn to use different codes because of our early life experiences, or because of falling off the swing at preschool, or maybe the codes change from being happy to being sad or from young to old, night to day. Who knows? Well, I'll tell you somebody who will never know: the biological reductionist peering down his microscope.

The answer is that we cannot eliminate the mental component of our lives by reducing it to the physical substrate. This is not to say that the mind is not dependent on the brain, because it is, but it represents a different aspect of brain than the brain's glucose consumption or its catecholamine output. Given these logical objections, why would anybody bother with reductionism? The answer is fairly simple. The problem has always been that we have no tools for dealing with the mind in the scientific setting. Therefore, if mind can be reduced to brain, we could solve the problem because mind could then be investigated by the tools of ordinary biological science. How come nobody in Kandel's department has told him his program is logically impossible? I've never been there so I don't know, but I doubt you get very far in a prestigious academic department if you start telling the Nobel Prize-winning head of department that his program stinks. Criticism is the essence of science, except when your job's on the line.

The crucial point is not whether science is any good at answering questions, because it clearly is. The point is whether it can answer all possible types of questions: equally clearly, it cannot. Before applying the principles and methods of science to a particular question, we need to be sure whether the question has an empirical content or whether it is purely metaphysical. If it has no empirical content (such as "What is the genetic basis of being a Christian?"), then science cannot answer it *in principle*. The inappropriate application of scientific principles and methods to questions of no empirical content is called **scientism**. Scientism is a grave error. Kandel's brand of wildly optimistic and completely unarticulated "radical reductionism" (his term) is pure scientism, and is therefore a grave error. It cannot achieve his goal of explaining "...perception, learning, memory, thought, consciousness, and the limits of free will."

So much for biological reductionism; shall we move on?

* * *

As we survey the gloomy landscape, littered with the wreckage of a hundred models that didn't fly, what is left? The latest cab off the rank is known as **functionalism** and, as the name implies, it is both clever and difficult to grasp. The best-known functionalist is the Boston philosopher, Daniel Dennett, although he has moved away from it a little in recent years and now attends more to philosophical aspects of evolutionary theory. Nonetheless, he is a prolific writer of books which quickly jump to the top of the academic best-seller lists – quite an achievement for a philosopher. Now approaching his seventies, and not in robust health, he maintains a punishing schedule of lectures, conferences, TV shows (you can find him on Youtube), books and papers. I've devoted a lot of time on Dennett's theories and, for full details and references, you should see Chap. 9 of *Humanizing Madness* (2007) and Chap. 1 of *Humanizing Psychiatrists* (2010).

Dennett is certainly not shy about his position. It is the clearest possible statement of materialism: "The prevailing wisdom... is materialism: there is only one sort of stuff, namely matter - the physical stuff of physics, chemistry, and physiology - and the mind is somehow nothing but a physical phenomenon... We can (in principle!) account for every mental phenomenon using the same physical principles, laws and raw materials that suffice to explain radioactivity, continental drift, photosynthesis... Somehow, the brain must be the mind."

Let's start with the beginning. His theory of mind, or of consciousness (he uses the terms interchangeably), is bitterly, even fanatically antidualist. He loathes and detests dualism as a feeble pseudo-explanation of what minds are all about, fit only for the rubbish bin of history. In fact, his dislike goes back a long way, to his first days at college in the very early sixties. Since then, he has elaborated a model of mind which fits in the functionalist camp. *The Cambridge Dictionary of Philosophy* (1995) defines functionalism as "the view that mental states are defined by their causes and effects." Hmm, that's not immediately apparent, but they continue: "What (qualifies) an inner state (as) mental is not an intrinsic property of the state, but rather its *relations* to sensory stimulation (input), to other inner states, and to behavior (output)." That is, if we want to explain the inner state of, say, being hungry, as a mental state, we don't try to explain the *experience* of being hungry, because that goes nowhere. Hunger is an intervening state between low blood sugar and reaching for food but there isn't something about the experience of hunger as such which makes it a mental state. Got it? Well, nor have I. Functionalists are not so much trying to *explain* hunger as they are trying to *explain it away*. They are saying: "We can't actually deal with this peculiar property called mental, but you don't have to worry because it's not what you think it is. We can explain everything without invoking it." If that sounds a bit like the behaviorists, don't be surprised, because it was their ploy, too.

Functionalists give the example of being in pain. Forget the mentality of pain, they say, it is actually the inner state caused by pinpricks (the input), which causes other inner states, such as worry (or anger), and then causes behavior such as saying "oh dear" or slugging the person who caused it. So, you may ask, how does that give us the *mentality* of a mental state? Well, it doesn't, of course, but that was never their intention. The intention was to glide over the mere mentality of mental states, in order to specify them better in the brain's economy and thereby avoid the trap of identifying a mental state with a brain structure (as MBIT tried to do, and failed). In this sense, it is an advance on reductionism and other forms of monism because it splits the function of mind from the physical structure of the brain, but therein lies its fatal flaw.

Several things emerge fairly quickly from this rather slippery attempt to explain mental states without mentioning that they are mental. Firstly, it is clear that, by this definition, a computer could have a mental state. We can program a computer to print "ouch" when somebody does something unpleasant to it (like accidentally press the esc button), or to voice certain naughty words and then lock the user out for ten minutes. That's all humans do, behaviorally, because unless we are the person who gets hurt, observable behavior is the only evidence we have that the victim has, in fact, a mental state called 'pain.' It also says that animals have pain states. With the functionalist definition of a mental state, it would be impossible to argue that animals don't feel pain or terror as they are slaughtered and that their mental states are of the same order of nature as ours. So it breaks down the barriers between humans and animals that, wittingly or otherwise, Descartes helped build years ago.

Second, being in a functional state called pain somehow seems to miss the point of the very painfulness of pain. The whole point of pain is that it hurts, and being in pain is something very different from pretending to be in pain, or being tickled. A large part of psychiatry is directed at distinguishing between people who claim to be in pain or sick or depressed, etc. from those who *really are* in pain, sick, depressed, etc. I have actually heard a doctor say to a patient: "You're not depressed, you only think you're depressed." Sort that one out in functionalist terms. School teachers may say (or they used to when I was in junior concentration camp): "He's not frightened, he's just talked himself into it." The question of what is the mentality of a mental state is not trivial. There is a huge industry out there of people cheating various insurance schemes (e.g. the gigantic industry for veterans or workers to get benefits they are not entitled to), nearly balanced on the other side by an industry determined to prevent people (such as veterans or workers) getting benefits they are entitled to. It would be so nice to be able to stick a probe in somebody and say, "Oh, yes, your back hurts to 13% only, so you can't get a pension," or to say to a soldier: "The scan says your bad dreams are driven by your unhappy marriage and your boozing, so off you go." Could there ever be a scanner that could tell when people are lying, or are fooling themselves or making themselves sick over nothing, or hiding genuine symptoms through embarrassment, and so on? I don't believe so, but a functionalist couldn't tell it, either.

The third complaint against functionalism is very brief: it is not a monist theory at all, it is simply the ancient hand of dualism hiding in a slick new puppet. Daniel Dennett is not a monist, he is a closet dualist. I think this is why he has given up on the philosophy of mind and taken up evolution, because his monist theory doesn't actually work. He hasn't any idea where it has gone wrong, meaning he can't fix it, so he has left the philosophy of mind to his students and wandered over to see what's happening in philosophy of evolution. They're fighting words if ever I heard them, so let's look at the details. The reason to look at the details is so you can see how analysis works (which will also let you know whether I'm right).

Dennett explicitly states that his work is a materialist theory of mind or consciousness, meaning he has set himself the task of writing a theory of mind that does not stray from that narrow cantonment in which the scientists play (always check the meaning of words. Cantonment means a designated area in which a group such as an army is confined. The operative word is 'confined' but it is not a prison; they agree to stay there but they could get out if they wanted to; sake for scientists). Now, if he says he is going to write a materialist theory of mind and he loathes dualism, that can mean only that he is going to write a monist theory of mind, i.e. one which is confined to the natural world of matter and energy but which explains *everything* about humans, such as pain, memory, intention, personality, etc, in matter-energy terms. Hmm, this is quite a program. Maybe he should have stuck to nuclear physics, it's easier.

The first step is to exclude reductionism. Functionalism is not a special case of reductionism because the functionalist would never claim he can reduce a mental property to its physical substrate. Mental properties are not to be found in molecules. They may be a property of clusters of molecules acting in a certain way but molecules don't hurt. Thus, functionalism is a special case of what used to be called **emergentism,** meaning the idea that complex behaviors and properties emerge as a structure becomes bigger and more complicated. The functionalist says that any mental property, meaning mental state, can emerge if the wiring is right. Dennett explicitly states that all the properties of tasting a wine could be duplicated on a microchip, and then the experience would emerge, too: "If all the control functions of a human wine taster's brain can be reproduced in silicon chips, the enjoyment will ipso facto be reproduced as well" (*ipso facto* means 'by that very fact,' and thence inevitably). Reproduced, emerge, same thing. This goes back to a 17th Century philosopher named Baruch Spinoza (until he converted to Catholicism at age 22yrs, after which Baruch became Benedict). He talked about dualism in a special sense, where the new property emerged, i.e. **property dualism.** Things can have different *properties*, but that doesn't imply *substance* dualism. I think this point is very important and will come back to it.

So the functionalist mind is very definitely a product of the material world: look at Dennett's stance again: "I declare my starting point to be the objective, materialistic, third-person world of the physical sciences..." No room there for equivocation, Prof. Dennett is a man of the dirt. So where do the mental properties that we are trying to explain fit in with "...the physical stuff of physics, chemistry, and physiology... radioactivity, continental drift, photosynthesis..." What is the *Somehow* in "Somehow, the brain must be the mind"? His answer is simplicity itself: that marvelously complex machine (Descartes again) called the brain is controlled by a virtual machine. That is, the brain generates a special sort of machine that can switch from one phase to another at blinding speed to make the decisions that we need to recognize a pinprick and say 'ouch.' But it's not just any old virtual machine, it is capable of generating more virtual machines on the run. We humans have "...the kind of mind that can transform itself on a moment's notice into a somewhat different virtual machine, taking on new projects, following new rules, adopting new policies. We are transformers. That's what a mind is, as contrasted with a mere brain, the control system of a chameleonic transformer, a virtual machine for making more virtual machines."

So you see, he clearly distinguishes between the brain and the mind that inhabits it. The brain is a chameleonic transformer, an ultra-sophisticated physical switching device, but still a "mere brain" made of "...the physical stuff of physics, chemistry, and physiology... radioactivity, continental drift, photosynthesis..." On the other hand, the mind is "...a virtual machine for making more virtual machines" as it needs them. Now, given that he won't allow any talk of two systems of stuff in his model of mind, what does this actually mean in practice? His virtual mind does the "heavy lifting" of his theory; it is the extra bit that does what animal brains can't do. It talks and makes major decisions, it has free will and follows lines of inquiry to build nuclear power stations, to map genomes and write poems and declare war. In short, it is the bit of us that makes each of us a knowing, sentient "me" and not a zombie or a desktop computer. It is, as you will recognize, the bit that was left over when silly old Descartes cut off everything and deleted all the bits he couldn't be sure of, to arrive at the conclusion: "Il y'a toujours quelque chose, et c'est moi." (*That's* French. It means, "Hey, mum, there's something here, and it's me" but Descartes had culture, so he said: 'Cogito, ergo sum,' which is Latin for 'I think, therefore I exist'). That is to say, by twisting and turning heroically and putting physics and biology talk where other people used philosophy talk, Dennett ended up exactly at the point Descartes did, but 350 years later. Rather sad, isn't it. That's why I say Daniel Dennett is a closet dualist.

You don't follow me? OK, look at it this way. Dennett has said the brain can't control itself. Fair enough, the mere physical structure of a nuclear power station can't control itself either, it has to have a controlling element and that element is its computer system. Inside that computer system is a digital model of the station, meaning a *virtual* model of the power station. The computer also has a lot of subsystems that monitor everything happening in the station. As it gets the current operating data, it plugs them into its *virtual* model of the station and then computes what its short and medium term future state is likely to be. On the basis of those computations, it decides on any changes it has to make to keep the whole show running smoothly (the Chernobyl disaster occurred because the human operators switched off the station's self-controlling systems to run a disaster simulation. Truly. The Stuxnet virus first recorded the normal operating data of the centrifuges, then sent them into overdrive but it fooled the controls in the operating system by feeding it the pre-recorded normal data). But the crucial point is that the digital model and the control systems in the computers are not real. Most emphatically, they are *not* "...the physical stuff of physics, chemistry, and physiology... radioactivity, continental drift, photosynthesis..." They are not these things *just because* they are virtual. That's what virtual means. To rephrase that, electrons and other physical things cannot, at a moment's notice, generate more electrons. They can't do it *just because* they are of the physical realm, otherwise we would breach the laws of thermodynamics. Virtual machines, however, most certainly can and do generate an infinity of virtual machines *just because* they are *not* part of the physical realm, so there's no breach of fundamental laws of physics.

Now some people are inclined to argue with this, on the grounds that the digital model arises in a physical system, therefore it must be physical itself, but this does not follow at all. Virtual does *not* mean physical. Virtual means *not* real, it means *not* of "...the physical stuff of physics, chemistry, and physiology... radioactivity, continental drift, photosynthesis..." The word virtual, on which hangs Dennett's entire life's work, just means (where's that dictionary?) let me see, Virtual, adj. Having the essence or effect of but not the appearance or form of.... Well, that seems pretty clear. A virtual machine is not the same as the real machine. You can ride a real horse but not a virtual horse. You can get fat on a real meal but not on a virtual meal. And if I pay my bill to you with virtual money, you might be annoyed unless it is the sort of virtual money that comes on a credit card. So there is the definition: a virtual machine is most assuredly *not* of the same order of being as a real machine. It is something different, of a different nature, maybe doing the job of but not having the same form as a physical machine (like the brain).

If anybody doubts this, then let me take a pot shot at you with my rifle. In fact, I've got two trusty rifles, one an antique I bought many years ago and the other quite new. The antique is heavy, over 1.5kg, and packs a wallop. Anything hit by that doesn't get up in a hurry. I've also got a virtual rifle. It weighs nothing, has no shape or color or smell, and it can't even be found but it lives in a computer and I can use it with a mouse to kill virtual grizzly bears which live in the virtual woods in my study. Which one would you prefer me to shoot you with? Thank you, I knew common sense would prevail.

So now everybody agrees: virtual is different. Therefore Dennett's claim that "Somehow, the brain *must* be the mind..." fails the critical test of monism in that the mind, as a *virtual machine*, cannot be the brain, which is a *real machine*. Therefore, he has invoked a dualist system and, therefore, all his ranting and raving against Cartesian dualism (and he has done a great deal of ranting and raving about it) amounts to naught.

The hard work in his model is done by something which is most assuredly *not* of "...the physical stuff of physics, chemistry, and physiology... radioactivity, continental drift, photosynthesis..." It is something else. If you say on the one hand that the mind is a virtual machine and, simultaneously, that the mind is somehow the brain, then you are saying the virtual machine is somehow the same as the other physical machine, which is gibberish. All of this follows from Dennett's claims. It was all buried in his prior assumptions, in the nested beliefs which supported his, shall we say, *vigorous* antidualism.

For those who are interested, exactly the same problems are to be found in the philosophy of John Searle, who advocates what he calls biological naturalism. This is also based in a rigid and uncompromising antidualism: "I think (dualism) is false..." "I do not believe that we live in two worlds, the mental and the physical... dualism in any form makes the status and existence of consciousness utterly mysterious... Having postulated a separate mental realm, the dualist cannot explain how it relates to the material world..." "The way to defeat dualism is simply to refuse to accept the system of categories that makes consciousness out as something non-biological, not a part of the natural world." "Above all, consciousness is a biological phenomenon. We should think of consciousness as part of our ordinary biological history, along with digestion, growth, mitosis and meiosis." Elsewhere, he adds photosynthesis and the secretion of bile to this list, leaving no doubt where he stands: "We live in one world, and all the features of the world from quarks and electrons to nation states and balance of payments problems are, in their different ways, part of that one world."

That's all fairly clear, so what does he propose for his monist model of mind? "All of our mental phenomena are caused by lower level neuronal processes in the brain and are themselves realized in the brain as higher level, or system, features." The mind is not, however, an ordinary biological phenomenon like, say, "digestion, growth, mitosis and meiosis, photosynthesis and the secretion of bile." No, "...consciousness is caused by brain processes and is a higher-level feature of the brain system." Now that term "higher-level feature of the brain system" is the give-away. It is the weasel term, the slippery "let's have a dualist mind when we're not having a dualist mind," expression that wrecks his theory. This is because a "higher-level feature of the brain system" is not itself a part of the physical brain. It is different, a property or performance of the brain but not the brain itself, just as high-C is a property or performance of a larynx without being the larynx itself. Thus, you see that Benedict Spinoza got there 300 years before Searle.

Searle's mistake is this: because of his visceral antidualism (which he shares with Dennett, so it must have been a product of their era because today's young people don't have it), he could not see that something that arises from a physical machine (call it a higher-level feature, or maybe even a virtual machine, it's the same thing) is not thereby a physical thing itself. It may be an informational thing. And, if it is stored in the right computer and connected to the right peripherals, information can certainly move mountains. Information, and the physical machine that stores it, are not each of the same order of being. They are a *dual* system, i.e. Searle also invoked dualism to save his monist system. His error was to confuse the provenance of a higher-level system (meaning its origin, the physical machine itself) with its ontology (meaning its nature).

That's enough on monist models of mind. I do not have any idea as to how a machine and its virtual or higher-level control system can be of one and the same order of being. Maybe that's just my failure of imagination but I prefer to blame the older generation: it's *their* failure of imagination. They just can't see how information runs the universe, and that an information system is ontologically distinct from the machine in which it is running. Dennet hinted at this with his example of the wine taster on a computer chip, but he couldn't reconcile information with physical machines, so he wandered off to see what was happening in the philosophy of evolution.

* * *

As you can see, dualist models of mind have been getting a lot of bad press from people pushing the monist barrow but, at this stage, it looks as though monism has run out of options. I now see them as the product of an age, i.e. people were disgusted with the excesses of the mentalism in psychoanalysis and also with the time-wasting of introspectionism. At the time, it was reasonable for the notion of monism to be explored, but it didn't work out. People leapt madly off an intellectual cliff, convinced that they would have a soft landing but they haven't had a landing at all. Neither Dennett's nor Searle's monism has had anything to say about mind-body interaction, mainly because they didn't see it as a problem. If mind and body were each of the same stuff as neurons, bile, photosynthesis and bone, then how could there be a mind-body problem? They tried to legislate the problem away: "We, the assembled senior philosophers of the generation of 1940, hereby decree that the mind and the body are of the same order of nature, so there can't be a mind-body problem and anybody who says there is won't be allowed to come to our party, so there."

However, in 1977, there was a flurry of sedition in the camp. Somebody dared to publish a book which was frankly dualist in nature. And not just anybody, but two bodies who definitely were somebody. For two weeks, two elderly knights of the realm, Sir Karl Popper and Sir John Eccles, a philosopher and a Nobel Prize-winning neurophysiologist, sat in a villa above a Swiss lake and talked about the nature of mind. From it came a fascinating but ultimately disappointing book which attempted to show that a non-physical mind was essential in attempting to explain human behavior, and how such a mind could interact with the body. In the first part of the book, Popper tried to show why mind-body interaction was necessary, and the metaphysical form it would need to take. The second part belonged to Eccles. He invoked a frankly religious or supernatural Self which interfered with the brain to "read" the cortical modules and make the myriad decisions we need to survive the day. It didn't work. For reasons I have outlined in Chap. 4 of *Humanizing Madness*, they were unable to achieve their goal. Their failure was not a problem of more time at the lake or more money, the error was conceptual. They could no more solve their problem than they could be in two places at once, i.e. their approach was logically impossible.

They had a history. Popper was a Jewish refugee from post-*Anschluss* Austria (look it up) who had gone to England but was unable to get the work he wanted and was also in danger if the Nazis invaded. Finally, he was appointed to a post in New Zealand, where he had a very peaceful war. After the war, he met Eccles, an Australian who was then a rising physiologist working in New Zealand for a few years. Post-war, Eccles had a brilliant career, culminating in sharing the Nobel Prize of 1963 with Hodgkin and Huxley. He was a devoutly religious person throughout his life and didn't like the rabidly reductionist materialism that was so popular with American psychologists and communists. Popper also despised communists and psychologists in roughly equal measure, so his and Eccles' collaboration was a natural. The problem was they were coming at the question of mind-body interaction from opposing points of view. As a physiologist, Eccles simply did not believe that the brain and the neurons he saw in his daily work could account for such complex matters as religion, politics, science and art. He desperately wanted the religious soul to play the vital part in our mental lives. Compare this with Kandel, who has also spent his life peering down microscopes (and also appears to be religious) but who comes to the exact opposite conclusion. Same evidence, same motivation, diametrically opposed conclusions. So that just goes to show you cannot accept an opinion on the authority of the person making it. Popper, on the other hand, didn't have a religious bone in his body, so they were actually trying to achieve the same end for different motives and it didn't work. Good try, next please.

After their effort flopped, the dualist camp kept very quiet for a long time. In the early 1980s, the philosopher Mario Bunge bemoaned the failure of Popper's and Eccles' effort and wondered when somebody would make a decent attempt at a dualist model of mind-body interaction: "The great dualist counter-attack (to psychological reductionism) has yet to come," he complained. It was a long time coming, but come it did. In 1996, David Chalmers published *The Conscious Mind: in search of a fundamental theory*. His point is that the conscious mind arises from the natural substrate of the brain but by a law-like process of supervenience. It is not a random or unpredictable matter. Given the particular properties of neurons (as data processors) and the unique structure of the brain and its associated sensory and effector organs, then conscious experience was going to happen. He is explicit: mind and brain are definitely not one and the same thing. Yes, they are intimately related, to the extent that, if the brain malfunctions even slightly, it will have immediate and quite profound mental effects but no, the mind is ontologically different from the brain substance:

"...the real problem with consciousness is to explain the principles in virtue of which consciousness arises from physical systems." This is essential as he wishes to remain within the limits of the material realm. Mind and body interact by psychophysical laws which we do not yet know, but there is nothing supernatural about them.

To a large extent, this is promissory materialism again: Science will deliver the psychophysical laws governing the emergence of mind and those laws will also explain mind-body interaction. Well, that's comforting, but can we have an idea how long we will have to wait? And can we have some indication of how they will actually interact, as distinct from the fine promise that they will? No, no, on both counts. Chalmers is not a neurophysiologist; unlike the eternally optimistic Dennett, he doesn't even bother to pretend he knows his glabrum from his putamen. Herein lies a problem, because it would seem that the emergent informational state (the mind) will be determined by the structure and function of the brain. Therefore, only a neurophysiologist could answer the questions of How long and What form? Perhaps Kandel was right after all? Unfortunately, I don't think so.

The point about any informational state is that it is *not* dependent of the physical machine generating it. Any computational process is what they call *multiply realizable*, an ugly term meaning it can be realized or brought to life on multiple platforms (I think that's the jargon). I can compute 2+2=4 on any number of proprietary or generic computing systems, there's no limit. The essential point is that, until we know the codes the platform uses, we can have no idea of the rules by which it is running. Of course, we know one rule (that 2+2=4) but we don't know if that was a one off, lucky shot or whether the system actually does have a general rule for arithmetic computations. In the case of the emergent mind, the whole point is that we need the rules *before* we can have any idea of the exact nature of mind. Hmm, seems to be the end of the road for Chalmers' natural dualism.

I think there is a way around this problem. Remember I said the farmer doesn't care about his actin and myosin, all he wants is that he can lift the spare wheel and put it on his tractor. This is also true for the lady driving her little car around the city; as long as it goes and obeys the *general* rules of the natural world as she knows them (i.e. it is not a Harry Potter car with a mind of its own), she doesn't care what goes on under the bonnet. The same goes for the mind. It isn't crucial that I know how you compute 2+2=4, as long as you get it right each time. As long as the rules governing my computer's operations run properly, I don't need to know them. As long as my mind correctly computes anger, or flavors, or brilliant poems, I don't need to know what the rules are. I can get by with *general* rules of a form similar to the lady driver: "Oh dear, that dial is pointing low, I'd better get some more of that expensive stuff."

Therefore, I do not need the precise nature of the rules that my mind has used to compute a bout of depression, as long as I know the *general* processes. And the general process for depression is – generic loss. Any loss above a certain size will generate depression, with a reliability that allows me to say that if one of my patients is depressed, then he has experienced a loss. I can also say that, if the next man is feeling anxious, then he has perceived a threat somewhere in his environment. The trick for the psychiatrist is to find out where the threat is, as the patient may not know. Don't be misled by the biological psychiatrists who would claim: "Oh, no, depression *equals* a chemical imbalance of the brain." They don't have a theory or model of mental disorder that allows them to make that claim, as will be shown.

So, while I am using this computer, as long as I know that moving the mouse thus highlights a passage, and ctrl-X *means* cut, then I can get by comfortably. And as long as I can work out the generic rules by which a mind works (once it is in existence), I can get by comfortably. So, bearing in mind (*sic*) that people can tell lies, where do we work out the generic rules by which a human mind works? Simple. We go back to Africa where humans originated, and we watch the nearest cousins we have who can't tell lies. We do our field work on chimps and baboons. We soon work out that these amusing animals are actually pretty serious: those big teeth aren't just for decoration. We see that they are social animals who are highly territorial. Within their societies, they form dominance hierarchies, mainly determined by male competitiveness. They are xenophobic but also can be altruistic at times, but mostly only for those with whom they have social bonds. When threatened, they respond with aggression or fear, depending largely on their sex and where they are in the hierarchy. They have a sense of humor and can be very suspicious, where suspicion has high survival value but humor seems to be a "left over" disposition, i.e. secondary to something else but with no direct survival value of its own (like swimming is left over). They use tools and are capable of merciless attacks on their own or other species. And so on. We arrive at a set of general rules for one species, check them against another to get the general primate rules, then apply these to the peculiarities of *Homo sapiens*, i.e. that we have speech, opposable thumbs, and better intellectual capacity to draw rules from the environment and predict the future, etc. Other than that, we seem to be driven by our primate heritage a fair bit of the time (you can call our primate heritage human nature if you will, but it's actually higher primate nature). The arms race? Just a bit of male posturing coupled with human intellectual creativity. The fashion industry? Self-advancement up the sexual hierarchy. Obesity? You're joking, you can't work that out? Mental disorder? Ah, that's the interesting one, but it's another story.

As long as we know the higher order rules by which a system operates, then we don't have to know the actual codes that underlie the higher order rules. The purpose of having a philosophy of mind is to ensure that the rules we think we have found are in fact the rules that are doing the work, and not something else. If, as in biological psychiatry, we try to attribute all malfunctions in the system to physical defects (hardware, if you wish, or wetware in the case of brains) while pretending that there are no psychological (software) problems, then we will have missed a very important point about the human animal (as well as condemning multitudes of people to the wrong treatment). That point is that the beliefs and experiences of a human mind form one sort of reality, and any errors in that reality have to be corrected within it, not by devious means through another reality.

The human mind is a real, separate and causally effective thing intimately related to (in a causal sense), but ontologically distinct from, the brain. We are dualist animals. OK, we are animals with heaps of virtual machines in our heads. Just try to convince me that doesn't mean "of two separate orders of nature," which is the definition of dualism.

Chapter 3: Knowing

1. Epistemology

In a celebrated case in 1997, now known as the Norfolk Four, four young members of the US Navy, stationed at Norfolk Naval Base in Virginia, USA, were charged with the rape and murder of the wife of another sailor while he was at sea. They were convicted solely on the basis of their confessions: after interrogation, each man had admitted the ghastly crime and signed statements describing in detail the events of the homicide. Despite the violent and grotesque sexual nature of the offenses, no forensic evidence was ever found to incriminate them. Subsequently, another man whose DNA matched the crime scene, and who knew the details of the case intimately, confessed to the crime but insisted he had acted alone. Even though he was convicted of the same offense and sentenced to several life sentences, the four sailors were not released until 2010, and then only conditionally, i.e. the convictions stood.

During the 'Show Trials' of the Stalinist purges in the USSR in the late 1930s, impeccably patriotic senior members of the Communist Party and of the Red Army, including the Chief of Staff, Marshall Mikhail Tukhachevsky, were charged with treason. Inevitably, in each case, the defendants gave elaborate confessions admitting enormous crimes against the Soviet state, including plotting with the Germans to surrender during an attack in order to overthrow Stalin. They were all shot. In his speech to the Twentieth Party Congress, in 1956, Soviet Premier Nikita Khruschev revealed that the confessions were false and the executed men were, in fact, innocent of the charges.

In 1989, two electrochemists, Martin Fleischmann and Stanley Pons, announced that they had found evidence for nuclear fusion at room temperatures and pressures. Quickly dubbed 'cold fusion' by the newspapers, the announcement caused pandemonium in the scientific world. If it were true, it would transform human society (and not necessarily for the better). Soon after, the first doubts surfaced and, by the end of the year, cold fusion had been pronounced dead and buried by the skeptical scientific community. Needless to say, conspiracy theorists went into overdrive and a small group of people around the world remain convinced it is a reality but is being suppressed by the oil companies, who would be destroyed by such a discovery. While checking on those dates, I noticed that Andrew Wakefield's study linking autism to MMR vaccine has been declared a fraud by no lesser authority than the *British Medical Journal*.

These matters turn on the question: What can we know for certain? Related questions include: How do we know (anything); what is the difference between knowing and believing; what is the nature of belief; what amounts to justification or proof; what is the value of "evidence of the senses" if the senses are so unreliable; how do we lie, and so on. Questions of this nature belong to the philosophical specialty known as **epistemology**. They have been debated in philosophy since the beginning of recorded history, which tends to suggest they are not just critically important questions, but they are also very, very difficult. I am not qualified to teach epistemology, so I can only talk vaguely about it and hope to interest you enough to take it seriously.

In medicine, we are greatly concerned with establishing the truth of a proposition, such as: "In condition X, Drug A is better than Drug B." We have elaborate procedures to try to work through the many, many factors that may be involved in what seems to be (but rarely is) a pretty straightforward claim. Commonly, these types of claims are found to be biased, or based on the wrong evidence, or otherwise suspect. For example, in psychiatry, a lot of the claims relating to the efficacy of antidepressants were found to be based on incomplete evidence. When all the studies were incorporated, and not just those that had been published, the therapeutic value of antidepressants took a nose dive. What had been happening was that negative findings were simply not being published, so all the surveys were based on a biased sample of the evidence.

In daily practice, physicians are forced to grapple with some ancient questions, even if we tend to contract them to other people, such as drug researchers, or members of the Cochrane Collaboration. Let's look at a very common claim made by psychiatrists: "Mental disorder is actually a chemical imbalance of the brain for which drug treatment is the only rational solution, and failing to implement drug treatment is culpable." Actually, that is three separate but closely related claims, but it doesn't matter. Are they true? If you became a little ratty, would you like to be told you have a chemical imbalance of the brain and to take these horse tablets? Stripping away the notion of any moral issues in this type of claim, it is the case that no physician, or policeman, or nurse or fisherman or parent or citizen can afford to be ignorant of them: "What is truth?" That ancient question (or ancient curse) is still with us but, with issues such as global warming and nuclear warfare, and no vast New World to flee to, the stakes are immeasurably higher.

We have to start somewhere and, traditionally, thinkers have concerned themselves with the question of what constitutes the proper form of knowledge. Should we try to work out things from the beginning, arriving at a conclusion by a lengthy process of deduction, or should our knowledge be based on the hard evidence of our senses? The first is often called *a priori* knowledge, meaning starting at the beginning with first principles, and gradually assembling a structure of indubitable knowledge to use as the basis for daily life. It was hoped that this knowledge would be independent of mere facts, and therefore the more reliable. The second is known as *a posteriori* knowledge, meaning knowledge which comes after the event of an observed fact, otherwise known as empirical knowledge. As an example, mathematics is (mostly) *a priori* while biology is *a posteriori*. Unfortunately, *a priori* knowledge is too often contaminated by value judgments and even cheap prejudice, while everybody knows how easily it is to mistake facts, and how difficult it is to get two people to agree on the same facts. Compounding all of this is the (slight) human tendency to tell lies, especially when money or prestige are involved, and when aren't they?

The ancient world tended to be more concerned with *a priori* knowledge, and an example is the trouble Galileo had in trying to convince people that objects fell at the same rate, regardless of their size. His (alleged) experiment in dropping a musket ball and a cannon ball from the Tower of Pisa was not considered convincing by the powers that were. They had reasoned from the notion of teleology, that objects sought their natural position in the universe, and were satisfied that a heavy object would clearly be more inclined to rush to the center of the earth than a light object, so that was the end of the matter. The Eminent Authorities reached these conclusions after many years of solemn debate and consultation of the Scriptures and of the classics, but not by leaning over towers and dropping their balls. People who challenged them, such as Galileo was wont to do, were usually able to see the error of their ways after a call from the local branch of the Inquisition, as Galileo did.

To a very large extent, the blossoming of natural philosophy (what we would now call science) during and after the Renaissance represented a new willingness among the educated to look to the natural world for answers to their questions. Figures such as the anatomist, Andreas Vesalius, the astronomers Kepler and Copernicus, and so many other fascinating explorers of the real world, changed human society for ever. That is, they changed from trying to use "accepted principles" to work out how the world should be, to using observed facts to work out how the world is. Today, empirical science is dominant; the pride of rationalism, especially logic and mathematics, are now seen as tools of inquiry. Even logic itself has been handed to machines, no less, which can perform the most prodigious feats of logical analysis at the rate of teraflops per second. How amazing.

How humiliating.

Let's look at **rationalism** for a moment. If we start with no prejudices or preconceptions, using only the barest statements of fact, what deep truths can we devise about the universe? If you put it that way, not very many. The feats of intellectualism that were once seen as the peaks of human endeavor, tended to start with a very large number of undeclared assumptions, such as: "God exists. The Bible is the literal truth. We are right and everybody else is wrong. Off with their heads. Amen." Once these are removed, then the grounds for rationalism tend to shrink. For example, consider human rights. We would like to build a large structure of human rights but, if the individual, local, national and other assumptions are deleted, what's left? Surprisingly little. Human rights are not written on tablets of stone nor in the stars. They tend to represent the minimal agreements of the power groups and not much more. It is a matter of a group saying: "We agree that the following shall be deemed Human Rights, meaning anybody who breaks them will be in real trouble unless he has a bigger army or lots of oil." As you see, questions of knowledge quickly broaden to include questions of morality and other prejudices.

If we look at empirical knowledge, it is immediately clear that the room for error is enormous. In fact, there is so much error, fantasy and other nonsense that it is difficult to be sure of what we can be sure of. If we start with the evidence of our eyes, it is clear that people are routinely fooled by these most fallible organs. As every policeman knows, finding two witnesses of the same crime who agree on all the facts is a wonder. The other senses are no better and, capping it, human memory is notoriously fallible. Psychologists say that the further an event recedes in the past, the more likely it is that a person will be certain of his recall and the more likely it is that he will be wrong. So what can we trust? Well, quite a bit, actually. The whole point of the sensory apparatus is to keep us up to date with what is happening "out there," with some internal worries such as pain to liven things up. Our visual apparatus evolved on the plains of Africa, where there were plenty of neighbors who were alert and ready to take advantage of a little hominid who wasn't watching what was happening around him. Our eyes give an accurate picture of the world, accurate enough for us to pin our survival on them all day, every day: Can you see those stairs? Can you tell how fast that car is moving? Can you smell that piece of fish? It seems off to me.

We can conclude that our perceptual apparatus and our memory are good, but not perfect, so we use auxiliary methods of improving the odds. We get somebody else to confirm whether that is indeed a pink elephant next door or just the sun glinting off the trees; we write notes and keep records, we examine things from different points of view and, above all, we set up competitions in which academics challenge each other to prove their point. That is the most devastating of all and it brings out a crucial point: that certainty of knowledge is relative, but the odds are vastly improved if everything can be challenged. We no longer allow churches or mosques, political parties or pressure groups to set the scientific agenda, unless it is stem cells in the US, evolution in Iran or AIDS in South Africa.

One aspect of the question of knowledge that should be mentioned is loosely titled skepticism. A **skeptic** is a person who habitually doubts the authenticity or value of received or generally accepted truth. A skeptic is not a cynic, a person who sees ulterior motives or deception behind every action and who believes the worst about people or events. A cynic would say of a charitable person: "Huh, everybody knows he's only buying approval." The skeptic would reply: "How can you be so sure? How can you trust what other people say about him? How can you trust your own interpretation of his actions?"

Skepticism seems to appear in the human animal some time in adolescence, when the verbally clever youth learns that he can play the game, too. There is only one rule: Whatever anybody else asserts as true or reliable, jump on it and demand the proof.

When they give it, find fault, question, denigrate and otherwise have a good time at their expense. This is very popular among first year university students, especially if they are away from home for the first time, but we are pleased when they grow out of it, ideally (but rarely) in the first semester. It is much more common among humanities students than engineering and science, and often reflects their exposure to a particular teacher who habitually questions everything and everybody in this manner (and wonders why he can't get a better job than his stupid university). First year science students tend to rely more heavily on rote learning.

Again, we can blame the Greeks for skepticism as a way of life, but skeptics didn't get very far as they tended to annoy the ruling clique and often found themselves outside the city wall – or nailed to it. Skepticism then had a break for a couple of thousand years as it wasn't popular with the Church, nor with the recent secular variants of their very successful business model, mostly known as Communist Parties, not to overlook the Nazis and assorted Fascists who were also quite cool toward skeptics. Skepticism only reaches its full flowering in societies with high levels of tolerance of dissent and high levels of wealth, sufficient to support small groups of utterly parasitic individuals who get their jollies sitting around in smoky coffee shops telling each other how the university authorities don't have a clue while trying to catch the eye of the new blond who is struggling with the coffee machine.

There are two forms, knowledge skepticism and justification skepticism. The extreme knowledge skeptic claims that we cannot know anything. The extreme justification skeptic, as you might expect, claims that no one is ever justified in believing anything. I am not sure I could slide a cigarette paper between these two stances, because it seems to me that they lead to each other in a circle. Be that as it may, the correct response to anybody who makes either of these claims is to ask whether he believes it, or why he feels justified in saying it, and then wander off to do something more constructive than listen to him, like sleep. The incorrect response is to stand there and argue the point, because that is all he wants. At the end, you will walk away frustrated at human stupidity and he will go home, satisfied that he has defeated yet another tool of the bourgeois state who has been trying to control his mind. The extreme skeptic just wants to argue, but he has nothing better to say. It is, in fact, one of the variants of the paranoid state, and a sensible person never argues with the paranoid.

Having said that, we need to strike a daily balance between gullibly accepting everything the newspapers dish up and foolishly rejecting everything. Wikileaks is a perfect example of why we should keep our wits about us (I'm waiting for them to release something I didn't know or couldn't have guessed) whereas the catastrophic epidemic of AIDS in South Africa is the result of one man (former president Thabo Mbeki) deciding there wasn't overwhelming evidence that HIV causes AIDS, and the green monkey idea was a conspiracy by the CIA to put black people down. As a result, about 270 times as many of his people have needlessly died of AIDS than died under the entire apartheid regime, but we won't mention that, either.

Thus, epistemology comes down to a matter of what can we believe; what should we believe; who and what can we trust, what is justified belief, what is the nature of belief and of evidence, and so on. It is endlessly fascinating – and infuriating. Life becomes a matter of constantly striving to find the nearest approximation of the truth, bearing in mind that there are no hard and fast rules, except this one: keep your wits about you. Anybody who claims to be sure of something probably has an ax to grind or is making money out of it. No professor is allowed to say to you, "This is the truth, do not question it" because that is a breach of the ethical function of universities. For example, if a professor of psychiatry says to you: "Mental disorder is just a special form of chemical imbalance of the brain," ask him for his evidence. He won't have any. Ask him, if you like, whether he has any ties to drug companies. The answer can be frightening. Better still, ask him for the name of the model of mental disorder he uses in his daily practice, his teaching and his research, and three seminal references that set out the theory as a series of testable propositions. You won't get an answer. You might get an invitation to try another medical school, or even the army but, as you wearily lug your new rifle around the parade ground, you can be sure that what you asked is exactly in the correct tradition of epistemology. So is ending up in the army.

We are all little epistemologists. If we weren't, our protohuman ancestors would have been gobbled up by the protoleopards several million years ago. That explains why our knowledge of the world is biased in favor of information that increases our chances of survival. We notice and remember dangerous things before nice things. This may help explain why mental patients can't really think of anything good in their lives. They've been so busy paying attention to the threatening stuff that they overlooked both of the pleasant things that happened ten years ago.

2. Tools of Certainty

For my daughter's second birthday, my wife made her a lovely party frock. It needed a petticoat, so mother took her to the shops to buy one. She chose a pretty slip with lace and insisted on wearing it around the house. "Why are you wearing your petticoat by itself?" I foolishly asked. "It not petticoat," she replied firmly. "But it's got lace around the bottom," I ventured. She drew herself up with hauteur: "Not *every* dress wiff lace is petticoat," she announced with great dignity, thereby ending the debate.

You may not recognize it, but her statement was a perfect example of **logic**. It was the negation of the following proposition, which she detected I was using:

P: Every dress with lace is a petticoat.

Its negation is: Not P. In logic, this would be written: ~P. It would be read as:

Not every dress with lace is a petticoat, or: It's not true that every dress with lace is a petticoat.

The material implication is that there is at least one lacey dress in the world (and she was wearing it). Faced with such crushing (and valid) logic, I gave in and went back to blowing up the party balloons.

Negation is a **logical operator**. Logical operators are (wait for it…) operations we can perform upon propositions in a system of logic. It would then be a system of propositional logic, and all the possible propositions in that system would amount to its propositional language. How shall we define propositions? I'm not sure if anybody has managed to do so without slipping into circularity or begging the question, but you can all recognize a proposition when you hear one. It expresses a fact of some sort, even if it is buried in some attitude or disposition of the speaker's.

Examples of propositions include:

The US National Debt now exceeds 121% of its GDP.

Queensland is experiencing massive floods this week. (Next week, of course, that proposition may no longer be true but it is true this week).

I dislike sugary drinks. (This is a special case of a proposition. It is read as: It is true that I dislike sugary drinks).

An attack on our positions will constitute an act of war. (Bit risky, some people would say that events that have not happened cannot be classed as propositions because they cannot be deemed true or false. Get around it by saying: It is true that we regard all attacks on our… etc.)

Luke Skywalker was the son of Darth Vader. (Now it is getting sticky. It has the form of a proposition but what is the truth of its content? Get around it by qualifying it thus: In the fictional Star Wars series, the character 'LS' was the son of the character 'DV').

We could go on but you get the message. Sorting out true propositions from false propositions, from pseudo-propositions, ambiguous propositions, **truism**, etc., is difficult and important.

Now that we are (sort of) clear on what a proposition is, it will be apparent that propositions can stand in relation to each other.

The tree is big. The tree is green.

We define the relationship between the two propositions about the same tree as **conjunction**, or addition, and write it as follows:

The tree is big and the tree is green, or: The tree is big and green.

If P_1 and P_2 represent the two propositions, we write this as: $P_1 \& P_2$.

Propositions cannot be related directly unless they have the same referent or subject.

We could say: Mr Green is very fat. Mrs Green is gorgeous.

We could not say: Mr and Mrs Green are very fat and gorgeous.

Propositions are nominated by their referents and must not be confused, otherwise you get a failure of reference.

Logical operators define the operations that manipulate those relationships. *Negation* is the simplest as it is the only unary operator, i.e. it works on a single proposition. All the rest (such as *and, or, implies,* etc.) are binary operators. They place two propositions in the propositional language in a particular relationship to each other. Negation simply inverts the truth value of a proposition, i.e. if P is true, then the negation of the proposition is false, and if P is false, then negating it yields a truth. If the proposition that apples are delicious is true, then negating that proposition means that apples are not delicious, which is false. Simple. We do it all the time and, as my daughter showed, it may well be innate. She had certainly not been taught anything like logic but, by her second birthday, she intuitively understood that a statement could be inverted to yield something else.

It is said that there are sixteen logical operators but we can get by with about five at the most. As the child's intellect develops through its stages, the various operators make their appearance in a particular sequence. The Swiss psychologist Jean Piaget (1896-1980) charted these stages by studying his own children as they matured. His monumental work has since been confirmed and further elaborated and is now a major part of developmental psychology. Children cannot be expected to perform cognitive operations before they have the intellectual wherewithal, and this has had a substantial effect on the psychology and philosophy of education. Whereas my generation got a clip over the ear for making mistakes, the modern generation get a star for making the effort.

The purpose of formal logic is to facilitate our restless search for The Truth. A language consists of a range of different speech forms, if you like. The totality of human vocal communication includes laughter, incomprehensible teenage grunts and moans, cries of fury, tears and a whole range of articulations or misarticulations, even before we reach verbal speech. Actual speech itself includes questions, salutations and pleasantries, exclamations (obscene and otherwise), orders, emotional ventings, etc, before we finally get to propositions. Propositions themselves can be either false (including ambiguity and outright lies), universal truth (truism or mathematics), or specific truths. Even the latter can be further subdivided into metaphysical or empirical truths (*a priori* or *a posteriori*) (these are shown in diagrammatic form in Fig 8.3, Chap 8 of *Humanizing Psychiatry* 2009). It is important to be able to recognize each speech act for what it is. Most human speech is dross and quite a lot of human speech actually detracts from the sum total of human knowledge. But every now and then, perhaps by accident, somebody says something important that needs to be noted.

It is important to be able to recognize when a speech act is not intended to go anywhere, i.e. it does not express any valid propositions. Politicians in particular are good at this. They simply say the same thing over and over again, changing the emphasis or the word order and, at the end, everybody thinks something important has been said, but it hasn't (unless the politician slipped up). Academics are also highly qualified in the area of talking arrant but high-sounding nonsense, and the best example, one which is essential reading for every tertiary student, is Alan Sokal's brilliant hoax paper, "Transgressing the boundaries: toward a transformative hermeneutics of quantum gravity." This was published in the prestigious journal *Social Text* in the Spring-summer edition of 1996. I cannot recommend too strongly that every person engaged in any sort of serious intellectual activity (meaning all university students, if not their teachers) should read this case closely. It has generated a large secondary literature and shows no signs of going away, mainly because pretentious academic drivel shows no signs of going away (I have commented on this in more detail in Chap 4 of *Humanizing Psychiatrists* 2010).

If we strip away all the drivel and dross that people speak, we are left with a set of meaningful propositions of a form suited to manipulation by logical operators. It should be understood that logic is not so much concerned with the truth content of propositions as their relationships. As long as statements are in the form of "well-formed propositions," then they are suitable for a logical analysis, even if their content is nonsense. This is where it gets difficult. A logical system is as empty of content as algebra; indeed, some people say that logic just is a special case of algebra, or vice versa, it depends on who you ask. Logic also blurs across into the philosophy of language, to semantics and to more general mathematics.

That will have to do on propositional logic. It is a specialized field but the elements should be known to everybody with a nose for the truth. There is another form, sometimes known as informal fallacies in classic logic (i.e. reasoning, but not propositional logic), which is of considerable use to anybody who has to listen to contentious matters (that means all of us). This was probably what young Greeks learned to recognize in their rhetoric and debating classes a few thousand years ago, but the lessons will never go out of fashion. In all, there were some eighteen informal fallacies which you will still hear deployed more or less every day, mostly by people who should know better, or they do but are hoping you don't. These are not so much part of a formal logical system as rhetorical tricks or devices to pull the wool over your eyes in order to win an argument by foul means when fair won't do. Any person using them is not arguing logically, meaning he is arguing dishonestly. That is a sweeping statement but my defense is *noblesse oblige*: anybody in a position of authority has a duty to know when he is using any of the informal fallacies. If he doesn't, he is acting with reckless disregard.

Traditionally, they were divided in two groups, thirteen fallacies of relevance and five of ambiguity. The first group (fallacies of relevance) depends on the concept that the premises in an argument must be relevant to the conclusion.

1. Appeal to force (*argumentum ad baculum*): This is just an attempt to win the dispute by threats of force when intellect has failed. Sometimes, they can be very subtle; a claim that most people support an argument is little more than an appeal to force. It carries no weight. The fact that 90% of the population, or all wealthy people, or all educated, or all patriotic or all devout people etc. support a certain point of view, has no bearing on whether it is correct. A million educated people can still be wrong (but look out, sometimes they are right, too).

2. Argument against the person (*ad hominem* argument): This can either be direct abuse or denigration of the other side, on the basis that, say, anybody who has unpaid parking tickets can't be trusted. It also can be used to taint a person's case by showing

that he has a vested interest in the outcome. Both of these claims may be reasonable but that's not the point: an argument stands or fails not on the basis of who is making it but on its intrinsic worth. Politicians use *ad hominem* arguments all the time, as do lawyers. Lawyers will attempt to influence a jury by casting aspersions against the witnesses for the other side. There is a psychological basis to this. We prefer the people we like to be all good and the people we don't like to be all bad. It makes for an easier life. However, even our enemies are capable of telling the time correctly: the fact that we dislike them doesn't mean we can reject all their statements. If we do so, we are making what is often called the 'genetic fallacy,' i.e. rejecting some information on the basis of its origin (or genesis). Much as I may dislike somebody, it doesn't justify rejecting everything he says on that basis alone. There was a celebrated case in the US some years ago in one of those pre-election debates for the town dogcatcher or something. Right at the end, the frothing Republican stood and, quivering with rage and disgust, demanded of the audience: "I'll tell you something about this man. He is a pedagogue. Would you elect a pedagogue?" The pedagogue, more commonly known as a teacher, subsequently lost but, even if he had been a pedophile, he may still have made a good dogcatcher.

3. Arguing from ignorance, perhaps better known as 'absence of proof is not proof of absence,' and its converse: 'absence of disproof is not proof of presence.' The fact that no living person has seen a Paradise Parrot does not prove they are extinct, and the same fact does not prove they are still around. The fact that no living person has seen a flying saucer doesn't prove a thing. It doesn't prove they do exist but are never seen because ETs are smarter than the average human. It also doesn't prove that the government is suppressing the information. The fact that there are no cars running on water does not prove that the oil companies have bought the patents for water engines and locked them away (patents have to be registered, after all, and they also expire). It is the basis for witch mania and its modern variants. The only thing you can say is: "We do not have sufficient evidence to decide this question one way or the other. We need to look elsewhere to settle it." Arguing from ignorance is the stock-in-trade of the ardent conspiratorialist, which is also a variant of the paranoid personality.

4. Appeal to the people (*argumentum ad populum*, appeal to the mob). This is an underhand attempt to appeal to the emotions, meaning base instincts, of the audience. This can be done by using tendentious words (describing an invention as 'new-fangled' where the implication is junk) or by associating the case with famous people or places. Advertisers do this all the time by selling breakfast food as 'the food of champions,' makeup 'as used by all the rising stars in Hollywood' or putting advertisements for men's underpants in women's magazines using heroically endowed, sultry young men as the models. Glamor, wealth, youth, charm, sun tan, big muscles and/or big breasts will not come your way just because you eat Crunchy Flakes. Sorry.

5. Appeal to pity (*argumentum ad misericordiam*). This is probably a variation on appeal to the masses, but the debater appeals to the tender feelings of his audience, if

they have any: "I ask you, members of the jury, look at this poor, pathetic creature. His life has been one of abject misery and squalor since the day his parents abandoned him....etc." Yes, but he may still have murdered the old lady for her pension money. A subtle variation is "but wouldn't you have acted the same way?" You may have, but you didn't. That has nothing to do with the facts or with the law. He did act that way, and was caught. The law is pitiless.

6. Appeal to authority (*argumentum ad verecundiam*): This is the perennial favorite of law and medicine. I hear it all the time: "A Nobel Prize-winning neurophysiologist says that mental disorder is wholly a matter of chemical imbalances of the brain. Prof X and Prof Y, of the Sydney University Institute of Brain and Mind Research, fully agree with him. Who are you to challenge these eminent authorities?" The only answer, to be repeated patiently, over and over again, is this: When Galileo stood before the Inquisition, he faced ten of the world's most eminent intellectual authorities who forced him to recant. Yet who was wrong and who was right? (Can you name any of his judges?) Authority means nothing. All that counts is the nature of the argument and the evidence brought to bear on it. All authority passes away. Nobody is an authority for ever. Today's authority is tomorrow's has-been. Nobody is an authority on everything. Et cetera. Repeating this mantra is tiresome, tedious, and endlessly necessary.

7. Accident. It is not possible to devise a general rule for all possible events, i.e. there are exceptions to every rule, and they do not necessarily disprove the rule (the exceptions may be a special case of the rule). Each case has to be decided on its own merits. Sometimes, what seems to be an exception to a rule actually supports the rule when it is examined more closely. The converse is, of course, converse accident or hasty generalization: the fact that opiates are beneficial in this case does not prove they will be beneficial in all cases.

8. False cause (*Post hoc, ergo propter hoc*) One of the most important goals in any sort of scientific research is correctly assigning causation. This is also true of law, as the opening paragraph in this chapter showed: Some men were in the vicinity when a woman was murdered, therefore they became prime suspects, even though they had no motive and, in several cases, perfect alibis (like, being at sea. You would think that would be a water-tight alibi). The fact that event B follows event A does not prove that A causes B. This is one of the most common logical errors of all, where logic is the study of valid inference. It is not valid to infer that A caused B just because of their temporal relationship, which is the basis of the Latin name for this error: "After the event, therefore because of the event." In medicine, it is a common cause of error. We have designed elaborate protocols to avoid this, such as the double-blind cross-over trial for drugs, etc. If a person is given a drug and gets better, what does it prove? In the vast majority of cases, it proves only that he was probably going to get better anyway. It really comes into its own in psychiatry. If a person has a form of psychotherapy and gets back to normal, what does it prove? Absolutely nothing, but this is how

psychoanalysis arose, and a whole thieves' kitchen of pop psychotherapies, such as primal therapy, EST, Syn-Anon, rebirthing and so on. But the opposite is also true: If a person undergoes a form of treatment and seems to get worse, it doesn't prove he needs more therapy. It could and often does mean that the treatment is making him worse. There is powerful evidence to suggest that the management of mental disorders in the old, vast and inhumane mental asylums (that should be *asyla*, but nobody knows that these days) actually converted people with fairly brief and/or benign disorders into severe, chronically ill inmates. I am also starting to think that the reason the consumption of antidepressants, mood stabilizers and antipsychotics is rising remorselessly, just as the rate of diagnosis etc. rises, indicates that the drugs and the mental set of the psychiatric industry are the cause of the problem, not the cure.

9. Begging the question (*petitio principii*). Quite often, you will read something like: 'The prisoner said he didn't commit the robbery at the office but this begs the question as to what he was doing there.' That is wrong. It does not beg the question at all: it is a case of 'raising the question.' Begging the question is to assume the truth of that which requires proof: "The Aboriginal is an inferior type of person. We can see that because he is always dirty. If he were not always dirty, he could get a better type of job but he would never be happy because keeping clean doesn't come natural to inferior racial types." This type of argument tends to be confused with what is called a vicious circle: "Whenever I get nervous, I have to drink to calm myself down. But as soon as I wake up each day, I start to panic in case I won't be able to get enough grog to get through the day." That is different, because the person makes a prediction ("If I don't drink, I'll be a mess"), and then it comes true just because he has made it, i.e. a self-fulfilling prediction. Begging the question is often quite subtle. It is commonly seen in difficult topics where there aren't a lot of facts and passions run high, i.e. anything to do with crime and law, education, national defense and mental health. Essentially, your opponent believes X is Y, but he needs proof to convince you, so he casts around until he finds some sort of evidence, overlooking the fact that what he thinks is evidence is not true unless the conclusion is accepted. Let's consider a historical example: "Mentally ill people should be sterilized for the betterment of society. In the main, they do not oppose it, which only goes to show how depraved they are and how society will be improved by preventing them spreading their inferior blood." If, as a lonely, frightened, poorly-educated 21yo, you had the choice of spending your life in a lunatic asylum or accepting sterilization in order to get out, which would you take? In begging the question, the conclusion is assumed as truthful; all that is needed is some evidence, and any evidence will do, even if the conclusion caused it. If, in listening to an argument, you have the feeling somebody has just pulled a sharp one over you but you can't quite see it, it is probably a case of begging the question.

10. Complex questions. Lawyers specialize in this because they know it confuses people, especially well-meaning people, which tends to exclude most lawyers. The simplest type is use of tendentious language: "So are you saying that this awful man is a

psychopath?" If you say yes, it will be thrown at you later that you said he was an awful man. If you later object on the basis that they were actually the lawyer's words, not yours, you will be told: "Yes, but you didn't object at the time, did you." These are complex questions as they are loaded with hidden meaning. Ending a sentence with "did you?" makes the other person feel like a naughty child. Lawyers know this and practice sneering in front of their mirrors. Beware of the double-bind, in which there are two parts to the question but whatever you answer will negate the other part: "You're a very naughty boy but you know mummy loves you, don't you." If the child answers Yes, he is agreeing he is very naughty; if he answers No, he is daring to argue with his mother and therefore he doesn't love her. I once had a very long cross examination by a decidedly hostile barrister from Sydney (lawyers from Sydney think people from Darwin drag their knuckles on the ground). He needed me to agree with his tame specialist from Sydney otherwise his case was sunk. "Well, Doctor," he sneered (where doctor rhymes with turd), "Professor Smith from Sydney thinks my client has PTSD. You are familiar with the facts, are you not? Fine, so if two psychiatrists are both familiar with the same set of acts, and psychiatry is a science, they should come to the same conclusion, should they not?" He had left himself wide open: "No more so than two lawyers," I replied. The courtroom erupted in laughter, and he lost his case. He was used to slick but insecure professors assuring the courts that psychiatry is indeed a science. If I had agreed with that proposition, then I would have been compelled to admit the unstated element in his case, that a Sydney professor takes priority over a provincial psychiatrist. So the principle is this: Always make sure you are aware of how many propositions are buried in a question. It is cash in the bank for a lawyer to dump complex questions on you, loaded with hidden assumptions and double meanings. In giving evidence, or reading a difficult paper, always insist that each proposition should stand alone. That is the only way complex questions can be sorted and prioritized properly. It is worth noting that, in the US, when a bill is put before the president for signature, he cannot sign the bits he likes and reject the rest. He has to sign the whole bill or veto it outright, no half measures. Thus, politicians attach all manner of "ear marks" to valid bills to get their bit of "pork" through. It is the same principle as complex questions: the president should only be asked, for example, to sign the defense appropriations rather than also sign for a bridge across Lower Dogpiddle Creek.

11. Irrelevant evidence (*ignoratio elenchi*). My favorite. There is a well-known political psychiatrist in Australia who, every time he is questioned about the validity of his work, starts to talk about the poor, neglected mentally ill people huddled in doorways in the driving rain. Almost invariably, this has nothing whatsoever to do with the question, but it makes wonderful TV. If you ask a politician for more money for shelters for homeless people, he will start telling you about all the government is doing to prevent illegal immigrants, or how they recently passed a bill spending more money on veterans, or something, but he won't answer the question. If you ask why so much money is being spent on drug research and not on other forms of management, you will

be swamped with a barrage of accusations that you don't support mental health research. You may, or you may not, but that has nothing to do with your question. This is the principle behind the suppression of an accused person's criminal record during a trial: if the jury knew he was the sort of child who pulled the wings off beetles, they would be more likely to convict. The fact that he has committed dozens of rapes in the past does not bear on whether he committed this one: he may have, he may not have. When psychiatrists are asked to justify using such large doses of drugs, they will often start to talk about how terrible it is to have a mental disorder. That, of course, is totally beside the point of the question but most people find it hard to interrupt and tell the speaker to answer the question. When you are confronted with this, especially if there is an audience, it is helpful to listen quietly until the speaker finishes, and then say: "That's fascinating, but I didn't actually ask you that. Now could you please answer the question?" (by that stage, he will usually have forgotten the question). Quite often, people will tell you all the good things they have done, rather than answer why they haven't done what you asked or what they were supposed to do. You should let them ramble on and, when they stop, look up in surprise and ask: "Oh, you've finished? I thought that was just the advertisement." The principle is simple: a question should relate to one proposition only, and the answer to a question must materially address the point of the question, and nothing else.

12. Irrelevant conclusion (*non sequitur*). This means "It does not follow." It means drawing the wrong conclusion from the evidence: "Jones did not turn up for the match so I conclude he is a cowardly fellow." Actually, Jones is in hospital with a broken leg from trying to defend an old lady against a mugging. "Insulin coma treatment has proven remarkably effective in treating chronic cases of schizophrenia." This form of treatment, which involved injecting chronic schizophrenics with insulin until they had seizures, then running in IV glucose to restore them, was widely used in the Western world for many years. In 1938, the eminent British psychiatrist, Ian Skottowe, argued that the insulin drove extra glucose into their frontal brain regions which cured their delusion and hallucinations. In 1953, a young psychiatry registrar (resident) at St Thomas' Hospital in London, Harold Bourne, showed that it was pure artifact. The extra care and attention given the patients, and the expectation of improvement from the staff, produced a short-term improvement. When the patients relapsed, as invariably they did in the old asylums, they got more of the same. For a truly frightening historical review of psychiatric *non sequiturs*, read Robert Whitaker's *Mad in America*. If that doesn't scare you enough, start on his *Anatomy of an Epidemic*.

The fallacies of ambiguity are not so clear (almost ambiguous, you might say). They can be very subtle, in that they depend on using a word with two different meanings or senses in the same sentence or argument. The behaviorist, BF Skinner, did this all the time but he had the linguist Noam Chomsky on his case. Repeatedly, Chomsky had cause to say of Skinner: "If he intends this as a literal, scientific claim, then he is wrong, but if he means it as a metaphorical claim, then it is trivial."

13. Fallacy of Equivocation: this depends directly on one word having two literal meanings and using it in both ways at different points in the sentence. The best example is a mantra from a certain religion we won't name: "The end of a thing is its perfection; death is the end of life; therefore death is the perfection of life." From this arose a particularly nasty cult of suicide and homicide. It depends on an error, that the word 'end' has two meanings. Literally, the syllogism should read: "The final goal of a thing is its perfection" (trite, dubious but harmless); "death is the final event of life" (true but not enlightening); "therefore death is the perfection of life" (whoa, doesn't follow at all. I choose to live, thanks). It also forms the basis of a large part of humor. We expect one use of the word but the sentence unexpectedly depends on the other. Another common error is to suppose that a word will keep its attributes if it is transposed to a different context: "He's a fantastic footballer, so I reckon he'd make a fantastic politician." Note the difference between this and: "He's a handsome footballer, so I reckon he'd make a handsome politician." What works in one context doesn't necessarily work in another. This type of error is not uncommon in psychology and philosophy.

14. Fallacy of Amphiboly, or failure of reference, is common and often humorous: "She left in a flurry of tears and a hansom cab" (very old example). "I'll hold the stake while you swing the mallet. When I nod my head, you hit it." There was a sign outside the operating theaters of my training hospital: "All patients must have their rings covered by tape." The daily horoscopes are a good example; they are so vague that they could apply to anything. Politicians try to speak in amphibolous terms so that, if their plans go wrong, they can claim they didn't intend that, anyway. Religious cranks often speak like this because their thoughts are so woolly, they can't organize them. If you try to force them to speak clearly, you will be accused of lack of faith. If you draw some unexpected conclusions from what they say, you will be accused of heresy. It allows those who want to be convinced to believe they have heard something profound, while unbelievers lose interest and go out for a beer. Thomas Szasz uses the fallacy of amphiboly all the time.

15. Fallacy of Accent. The meaning of a spoken sentence can change quite dramatically depending on where the accent lies. "*Would* you talk to your son?" "Would *you* talk to your son?" "Would you *talk* to your son?" "Would you talk to *your* son?" "Would you talk to your *son*?" Sometimes, the accent just lies. (Fallacy of equivocation, if you didn't notice.) The advantage of this is that the speaker can later deny any intent to deceive: "Oh, you must have misunderstood me. It was taken out of context."

That should do. The informal fallacies have been around for a very long time but they show no signs of going out of fashion. There are more but I don't think there have been any new ones for a few thousand years. If you wish to avoid being fooled by people, you will need to be able to recognize them. I suggest you learn one each morning, and then try to find as many examples of it as you can during the day. It will only take about two weeks. At the end of two weeks, you will be amazed at how insightful you have become. Unless you keep quiet about it, at the end of three weeks, you will be amazed at how few friends you have.

Chapter 4: Philosophy and Science

Psychoanalysts claimed their theories were scientific. Marxists claimed their theories were scientific. Behaviorists claimed their theories were scientific. All those doctrines have vanished like the morning mist. When the leucotomy was announced (lobotomy, if you must), it was proclaimed as a gigantic breakthrough in the science of mental disorder. It has since gone the way of leeches, which were once thought to represent a science of therapeutics. Nowadays, we have domestic science, political science, sports science, social science, military science, retail science, management science and so on. The Nazis even had a racial science. What is this strange thing called science that everybody wants a bit of the action? What is its attraction, what is its power over people? When we look at all the dreadful things that have been done in the name of science, you really would wonder why anybody would bother, but still they come.

We should stand a long way back and have a cool, unhurried look at it just to try and sort it out. Perhaps we could start by finding out what is common to all fields that claim to be science, and then maybe look at what scientists do, how they work out what is good science and what is bad, and so on. By doing that, we would be looking more at the form of any science rather than its content. Taking a cool, distant look at the form of science is known as metascience, but we usually refer to it as the philosophy of science. The philosophy of science is not a science in its own right, but there could be several philosophies of science, in which case, by comparing them, we would end up with a meta-metascience.

In the introduction to this essay, I suggested you should read at least a short history of Western science, and preferably a longer history of human science. The Western story starts, once again, with those restless Greeks, who separated the abstract study of things from technologies such as metal-working and ship-building. Ballistics, as the study of moving objects, was separated from the art of building catapults for war. They focused their efforts on mathematics but weren't averse to a bit of biology as well. The ancient idea of the brain as the body's cooling system is probably Greek, as is the idea of four 'humors' or fluids as the basis of life (similar ideas pop up in other cultures, of course; theorizing about the unknown is a human attribute, not Hellenic). Other quintessential Greek ideas include concepts of evolution, of atomic theory and of materialism.

However, the old notion of science as something you do by looking at the world took a severe beating from the spread of the central idea behind the "religions of the Book," namely that the nature of the universe was fixed at its creation and all necessary information about the universe was to be found in "The Book." By contrast, for the Greeks, religion was a relatively private matter with no fixed dogma and no centralized priesthood. Neighbors could practice quite different religious beliefs just because they always had, or because they came from different parts of the country. This meant that there were no squads of "thought police" peering over everybody's shoulders and no neighborhood spies, as there were in most of the major religions. To a large extent, the spread of religion homogenized thought, imposing a uniform belief system on all under its sway. As institutionalized Christianity arose in the West, so independent thought and inquiry declined. The entire Western world, from the far eastern borders of what became Russia down to the Eastern (Greek) Christian lands of the Byzantine Empire, and across to the shores of the Atlantic, fell into a state of suspended intellectual animation. Upholding the Divine Mystery was more important than penetrating it.

During these "Dark Ages" (they were only dark in the west, not in the Eastern Empires or the Caliphate), if anybody had any concern for the phenomena of the world, he was restricted in the evidence he could use to answer his questions (i.e. to the Bible and the classic Greek texts) and to the form of his deliberations. More or less the only way he could advance knowledge was by use of the process of deductive reasoning, of which the Aristotelian syllogism stood as the exemplar. **Deduction** is a particular form of reasoning or inference, in which the conclusions of the argument are contained within the premises. That is, deduction leads to one answer, and one only, because the answer could not be otherwise. For example:

This animal is a dog;

<u>All dogs have four legs</u>;

Therefore: This animal has four legs.

(It is written with the second premise underlined and 'therefore' is usually omitted).

In the act or process of deduction, the items of information in the premises are joined in such a way as to lead inevitably to a conclusion which is not stated in the premises. The conclusion is at once novel, inevitable and correct.

***

This is how things remained for the better part of a millennium and a half until, in 1453, the expanding empire of the Muslim Ottoman Turks finally conquered Byzantium. Actually, it wasn't much of an effort on their behalf. The Eastern Empire at that stage was corrupt and effete and simply slid wearily under Turkish control. However, the new rulers had very strict ideas on idolatry, i.e. the worship of physical representations, so many of the libraries of the Empire were emptied and shipped west to save them. Thus, the west suddenly became home to ancient texts from classical Greek times that had long been forgotten. This happened at the time of rapid commercial expansion in the western kingdoms due, as much as anything, to the development of ocean-going vessels and better methods of preserving food. For example, in 1492, Columbus reached the New World while, in 1498, Vasco da Gama rounded the Cape of Good Hope and reached India. Money, technology and ideas began the intellectual ferment in Europe known as the Renaissance and, in this setting, scientific thinking broke free of the restraint of the Church. That is, people who wanted to know about the natural world were gripped by the revolutionary idea that they should actually look at it, as distinct from the old idea of reading "the authorities," i.e. the Bible and the ancient texts.

Throughout the sixteenth century, there were rapid changes as people realized there were, for example, many more lands and peoples, and vastly more plants and animals, than their teachers had believed. The first of the systematic observations placing the sun at the center of the universe were undertaken in northern Europe, and were soon reinforced by Galileo and his bothersome telescope. In England, the politically influential Sir Francis Bacon (1561-1626) devised a method for investigating the natural world. Now, generally known as Baconian Induction, this consisted of amassing more and more detailed lists of observations and drawing general laws of nature from them. **Induction** is another form of reasoning but it differs from deduction because the conclusion is not contained in the premises. An inductive conclusion is based, not on watertight reasoning, but on limited observations of the world. The student of nature attempts to draw general laws of nature based on a limited set of observations, i.e. to make predictions about future incidents based on an imperfect or incomplete data base. This is the case of the "Xmas turkey." A young turkey heard rumors that, one day, the sun would rise but would not set so, each morning, he awoke wondering if this would be that terrible day. One day, he decided that he had enough evidence to say that, yes, the sun inevitably rose and set each day and that this represented a general law of the universe. He rushed around telling all the other turkeys who were greatly relieved. Unfortunately for them, the date was December 24th.

Baconian induction held sway for a long time but its deficiencies, and those of deduction, gradually became more apparent. For example, in the case of the dog, people started to wonder how we could be sure that this was a dog, and how anybody could guarantee that all dogs had four legs; was a three-legged dog not a dog? That is, they didn't worry so much about the syllogism itself, because that was considered impeccable, but about the nature of the premises. If there was one three legged dog in the world, then the syllogism, and all of the structure of science that it supported, broke down. Bacon himself had listed four faults that stood in the way of perfect general laws. He called these the Four Idols, the first of which was the tendency of humans to see order where there was none, and was due to people allowing their preconceptions of the nature of things to dominate their observations. The second was their tendency to interpret things in line with their personalities, and their likes and dislikes (not so different from the first). The third was due to confusion in the use of language, where different meanings of words influenced the selection of evidence. The last was a direct challenge to the authority of the church, in that people allowed academic dogma to influence their observations and questions. We would now see these tendencies as examples of **cognitive bias**, how people habitually interpret neutral or novel events in accordance with their preconceptions.

The problem for Baconian induction is just that its data set is incomplete. If this were not so, if it were complete, then the natural philosopher (later, the scientist) would be able to formulate the precise law of nature without making a leap of faith. Needless to say, the universe isn't quite so obliging. Practically everything we do depends on our perception of what is likely to happen, based on our experience of what has gone before, but it can go wrong. Over the centuries, various people have tried to formulate rules for induction so that it can be as reliable as deduction but they have all failed. If we could set up the process of induction such that it could be completely reliable, then it would either not be empirical or it would not be based on incomplete data sets. Either way, it wouldn't be induction.

One of the world's greatest scientists, Charles Darwin, used induction but was very aware of its deficiencies, so he amassed huge empirical support for all of his work. For the open-minded, the mass of supportive information standing behind the modern Darwinian model is now overwhelming but that is not the problem with evolution. The problem is not the people who are perhaps keen to be convinced but those who argue (justifiably): "You have not accumulated incontrovertible support; therefore, I do not feel compelled by overwhelming argument to accept your case." Now the problem here is that this is disingenuous, meaning insincere, because the evidence is in support of a theory, and not a formal rule of nature. Theories, by definition, are never complete, and the evidence for them is necessarily full of gaps. Take another example, the theory of gravity. This is strongly supported by a wide range of evidence from many sources, but it is a theory nonetheless because it is still an incomplete explanation of the phenomena. Given that it is not overwhelmingly supported by the evidence, would the people who reject evolution, because it is an incomplete theory, also reject the theory of gravity because it is incomplete? Would they, for example, be prepared to buy shares in my company which hopes to patent the world's first anti-gravity machine? Just think how profitable it would be so join the queue, friends, and have your money ready. No? Well, how come you buy shares in creationism?

* * *

This leads us to the critically important question of the nature of a **theory**. At this point, it would be easier for me to declare this chapter finished and go to bed but so much depends on this question that we will have to soldier on. In brief, a theory is an intellectual exercise designed to make sense out of our incomplete set of observations of the natural universe. Humans are curious creatures; we need to know what is going on behind the scenes. On the one hand, we have a set of observations; on the other, we want to know why just that set of observations exists and not another, i.e. what is the hidden mechanism generating just those observations and no other? For example, in northern Europe hundreds of years ago, it was noticed that swallows, which skim the water of ponds and rivers, disappear during winter. Somebody decided that they must spend the cold season asleep in the bottom of the ponds, protected from the storms by the ice above them. That is a theory, a postulated mechanism to explain the observations. A more sensible alternative would have been that they spent their winters roosting in the thatch of the peasants' houses. However, nobody ever found them there, and they had no way of searching the bottoms of the frozen ponds (absence of evidence, you see), so the pond idea won. Why did nobody suggest they flew thousands of kilometers each year to warmer climates? Probably because nobody thought such small birds were strong enough to fly those enormous distances. We now know that they rely on storm fronts for assistance in their travel plans but nobody knew about storm fronts in those days. Until the advent of rapid communications, weather was, as James Gleick observed, just a series of local surprises. Without up-to-the-minute information, there could be no *theory* of weather. A theory changes observations from piecemeal to coherent by uniting them under a single, unseen mechanism. A good example was Pasteur's theory of germs. In one stroke, he united a huge mass of diseases into a single phenomenon, infection (the exact opposite, as you will see, of the current diagnostic process in psychiatry, which keeps expanding the list of diseases).

The principle behind any theory is that it is a *suggestion* (hypothesis, in science-talk) of an *unseen causative mechanism* which is *one dimension removed* from the observations themselves, but the evidence for the postulated mechanism is *incomplete or circumstantial evidence* only. A *supernatural* theory would say something like: "At this point, folks, God intervened with a miracle." A *scientific* theory is one cast in the tradition of western materialist science, i.e. the unseen mechanism must be couched in terms of the laws of the time-space continuum and must positively exclude any and all supernatural elements. In addition, there must be no unexplained gaps in the causative chain that are not potentially capable of explanation within the laws of physics. Thus, the idea of swallows spending their winters cuddled in little mud nests in the bottom of ponds was a perfectly rational, scientific theory. It just happened to be wrong (cf. HL Mencken: "For every complex problem, there is an answer that is clear, simple, and wrong").

This leads us to the next question: how do we choose between theories? Given two suggested mechanisms which seem to explain the observations equally well (sleep in the mud vs. fly south), which should we choose? Well, despite anything the **relativists** or **post-modernists** might like to say on the topic, it is not a matter of flipping a coin. The whole point about being a scientist, as Bacon recognized, is to separate human prejudice and foibles from the serious business of coming up with the correct explanation of things *as they are*. At this point, we will jump several hundred years of confusing philosophy, to come to the late nineteenth century and the early part of the twentieth. This was another period of remarkable intellectual development, in so many fields: mathematics, chemistry, physics, biology, astronomy, geology, archeology, anthropology and so on. While the progress of physics and chemistry affected most people's lives, they were not especially contentious because most people neither knew nor cared about the atomic theory of matter, or whether the ether existed. It is true there were many theories advanced at the time which flowered briefly and then vanished without a trace. These days, with the advantage of hindsight, we would class many of them as crackpot notions but, at the time, they seemed to make sense, just as ours do today (even though some of them will inevitably be proven wrong_.

As long as scientists regularly served up bigger steel ships or improved telegraphs, nobody was much concerned with their arcane theories. However, in one area, this was not the case: Darwin's theory of evolution. This provoked the most ferocious controversy, one which is still raging a hundred and fifty years later. Darwin's theory was very unusual. In the first place, it was based on massive and overwhelmingly detailed observations. Nobody could argue against his empirical observations, because they were nearly faultless. In this sense, he was a very good inductionist in the Baconian tradition. However, his observations went much further. They supported a theoretical account of speciation which, firstly, was of no direct value to anybody (not like the huge industries supported by chemistry), and second, it drove a stake directly into the heart of human self-perception. Not only was this perception derived from Church authority, but it also served to reinforce that authority.

At the end of the nineteenth century and long after, Darwin's work was widely accepted in the scientific community but remained under sustained attack outside (see the celebrated "Scopes Monkey Trials" of 1925, in the US state of Tennessee, in which a school teacher, John Scopes, was charged with teaching evolutionary theory, which was then illegal. Fundamentalists supported the prosecution on the basis that the revealed word of God, as written in the Bible, trumped any and all human knowledge). Slowly, it dawned on evolutionists that, no matter how much evidence they found to support Darwin's revolutionary idea, their opponents could always find fault, which allowed them to reject it.

At about the same time, in Vienna and other *mittel-Europa* cities, philosophers were increasingly concerned with the nature of theories themselves, and how to distinguish good theories from bad. In briefest terms, they decided that a good theory was one that imparted knowledge. Specifically, the propositions that comprised that body of knowledge had meaning insofar as they could be verified. The principle of verification stated that the meaning of any sentence just is its method of verification, which quickly sorted all possible sentences into two groups. On the one hand, there was the group of sentences which could be verified by empirical observation and, on the other, there was all the rest. "All the rest" amounted to the very large group of propositions or claims which had no empirical support, namely, the very large part of human knowledge which was considered metaphysical. The difference between scientific and metaphysical propositions was just this: metaphysical claims could not be verified but were accepted as an article of faith. They were therefore dismissed as meaningless by the group, who became known as the Vienna Circle of logical positivists (don't ask). They were fairly sure that this distinction was of real value in defining science.

It wasn't long before a younger Viennese philosopher who was not part of the group raised an objection. Karl Popper realized that some claims, put forward as perfectly sensible solutions to unsolved problems, were not amenable to verification, which meant that, in the tight sense of the Vienna Circle, they were not scientific claims at all This did not strike him as very sensible because, even at that relatively late stage, Darwin's theory of evolution really could not be verified. Sure, there was evidence supporting it but, for every item of supportive evidence, there was at least one, if not a deluge, of counter-claims: just ask the knuckle-dragging fundamentalists who were stamping around the Tennessee schools, making sure their little dears didn't learn anything too modern. The problem was partly practical, that the process of evolution took place over eons, and also partly theoretical, in that there was no mechanism known that could account for the genetic changes on which it depended. Impasse. That meant that, by the strict regime of the logical positivists, evolution was not a scientific theory. Popper's idea was that the criterion distinguishing science from non-science could not be just the method of verification of its claims, but that a theory must be open to verification in principle.

Thus, a theory such as "angels exist" was clearly open to verification and, therefore, was itself scientific. This troubled Popper greatly. The statement "angels exist" could only be verified by catching an angel but, if they were half the beings they were supposed to be, nobody would ever be able to catch one. He therefore excluded what he called "existential statements" from the field of science. An existential statement is something like: "There are angels," or "Angels exist." The form of these statements generate arguments (or research programs) that could have no end. Failing to catch an angel does not prove they don't exist. Theories, he argued, had to be in a form that allowed us to test them before we have wasted much time on them. However, a test which was positive provided no solid evidence because we would not be able to prove that it was a general truth about the universe. That is, we would never know whether the evidence was just a special case – or even random luck – rather than a general truth. On the other hand, a theory that *failed* a test *just once* told us something terribly important: that it was not a general truth at all. This discrepancy or asymmetry between the evidence that could be used in science gave him what he wanted, a reliable means of distinguishing between claims that were potentially of scientific value compared with those that could consume resources endlessly and go nowhere, just because they were metaphysical statements masquerading as empirical claims.

The criterion or feature he chose to demarcate science from non-science (otherwise known as metaphysics, meaning propositions accepted on faith) was that the claim was capable of being refuted. Metaphysical claims are of a form that can never be refuted (how can you prove that angels do not exist?). It further followed, he argued, that the process of science was one of proposing bold, highly unlikely theories and then submitting them to stringent testing to see if they could be proven wrong. If a theory passed all the tests, it moved to a "higher level," meaning it was no longer mere conjecture but it had some scientific standing. However, any and all scientific theories can be overthrown by new evidence, and this is how science progresses. Metaphysical theories are fixed and are not subject to criticism or revision so they do not advance or develop. He warned that we need to be very careful of theories which always seemed to be one jump in front of refutation, the "Yes, but..." mode. A theory can always be "immunized" against refutation by a constant flow of minor revisions and changes and this also represents non-science at work.

By this standard, is the theory of evolution capable of refutation? It most definitely is. If a new species suddenly sprang into existence today, with no evidence that it had evolved from a previously known species, then it would be fatal to Darwin's hypothesis. New species are discovered all the time but nobody has ever found one that didn't have relatives nearby or in the fossil record. Even the bizarre organisms that live in deep oceanic thermal vents have relatives in thermal springs on land. A case of backward evolution would also be severely problematic for the theory: if the frill-necked lizards that live in my yard suddenly started breeding baby Triceratops, the theory of evolution would be in serious trouble. Fortunately, evolutionary theory is now immeasurably strengthened by the new science of molecular genetics. We are no longer in the difficult position of not having an *"unseen causative mechanism* which is *one dimension removed* from the observations themselves." Agreed, it takes special scientific instruments to "see" genes at work but the instruments are simply functioning as extensions to our eyes.

***

What, then, is the difference between a theory and a model? In simple terms, a **theory** is a statement of an unseen generative mechanism which can potentially account for the observations. Starting with an undisputed observation, the theory is set out in the form of a series of inter-related propositions, and it proceeds from there. Each new proposition must follow from the preceding set with no conceptual gaps in the causative chain. Finally, a theory must generate testable predictions with real consequences in the material world. A theory is an idea; it exists in the form of words only. Mathematical theories exist in the form of functions.

A **model** is the instantiation of the theory in simplified form. The bare essentials of the theoretical statement are used to build a simplified physical representation of a machine that exemplifies part of the postulated mechanism. A model never includes all the elements of the theory, only the bare bones, as it were, but there must be a one-to-one relationship between the theoretical elements and the mechanisms of the model. Mathematical models are similar. They take the essential constructs of the theory (which may itself exist only in mathematical form) and show how they would interact in the real world by generating outcomes that can be compared with reality. A computer model of the weather is a good example of the instantiation of a mathematical model.

Thus, we have a *theory* of heavier-than-air flight consisting of a series of inter-related propositions, namely:

(1) Bodies of air moving at different speeds show different pressures.

(2) If the bodies can be separated by a movable physical barrier, then that barrier will be forced to move to the area of lower pressure, meaning the area of higher speed.

(3) If the lower pressure is on the upper surface and the pressure differential is sufficiently high, the barrier will tend to move against gravity.

A *model* of heavier-than-air flight uses the different speeds on either surface of a moving aerofoil to generate a pressure differential. This means the lower pressure is on the upper surface, so the aerofoil will generate lift: the rest is just a matter of balancing the forces of lift and gravity to produce a stable aerial machine. A model of heavier-than-air flight is a physical object that flies through the air – and crashes. This is Popper's point: our theories and their models are expendable. We can have a theory of instantaneous transport but we would use a mouse in a scaled-down model before testing it on a human.

Two other points should be mentioned. Firstly, there is potentially an infinite number of theories that can be devised to generate a particular outcome; in real life, we will only be interested in the few of them that can do it economically (**Occam's razor**). Second, and flowing from it, each theory can give rise to dozens of models that may solve the physical problem, but only one or a few of them may be successful in practice.

It is important to distinguish between a theory as a set of statements or propositions, and a model as just one working example of a simplified version of those statements. A theory of nuclear fusion says that, under suitable conditions of temperature and pressure, a plasma can form leading to fusion. A corollary to the theory indicates that magnetic forces can create those conditions sufficient to test the theory. A working model is devised which might produce fusion for only a few microseconds but it is enough to show that the plan has potential. Needless to say, these programs often acquire a momentum of their own. If nuclear fusion is needed to keep up with our increasing consumption of energy, perhaps the money would be better spent on finding ways to conserve energy, to reduce consumption instead of finding expensive ways to increase it. So there are usually different ways of achieving a single goal. The theory usually doesn't predict the outcome at this level, mostly because nobody thought of it.

Let's look at my own field, mental disorder. For an outsider, one of the most striking features is the stunningly complex jargon that psychiatry uses. This is overwhelming: nobody but a psychiatrist has a clue what it all means, especially as it seems to change as time goes by. In the past, psychiatrists talked 'Freud-speak,' which nobody understood, but now they talk the impenetrable language of 'DSM and brain-speak,' and nobody is any the wiser ("I used to think I was anal retentive but now I've got OCD"). However, there is a problem for medical students in that nobody ever talks of an actual model of mental disorder. Needless to say, students do not notice this as, in their brief careers, nobody has ever talked to them about models of anything. Starting in school, and then in university, they have been drilled in a single approach to knowledge, one now called **reductionism**. The peculiar point is that not one of their teachers has ever explained to them what reductionism is, and the reason for this omission is simple: not one of the teachers knows, either. So perhaps we can finish this section with a brief look at reductionism and its application to mental disorder.

If we have something big and complex to explain, the usual method is to take it to bits. That is, we reduce it to its parts and show how they relate to each other, then we put it back together and, hey presto, it works (mostly, except for the bits left over). In Western science, this is universal, but not by accident. The whole point of Western science is that it is concerned with the matter-energy relationships in the universe, and the proper way to understand matter-energy relationships is to see how energy and matter move each other by virtue of their physical structure. Any machine, no matter how simple or complex, has a static physical structure, with inputs (of matter and energy) and outputs. We can track the inputs through the machine, as they move, combine, separate and recombine in different forms to produce the specific output of that machine. Without much effort, we can work out exactly what is happening at any particular time and, more importantly, we can then predict what will happen in the future. We do this by detailed understanding of the matter-energy paths within the machine. For example, the internal combustion engine in your car cannot produce an output of eggs from an input of kitchen scraps, even though a chicken costing a few dollars can. Similarly, the chicken cannot carry four people at 120km per hour for four hours. The thermodynamic relationships defined by the chicken's workings are of the wrong order to achieve this goal. A machine, be it a human artifact or a biological machine such as a yeast cell, can do only what its physico-chemical pathways permit. The job of a reductionist scientist is to understand, in minute detail, the contribution of each of the pathways to the final output. In ontological reductionism, we are mapping the precise matter-energy interactions throughout the machine because these specify the output.

There is no lower limit to reductionism. The properties of a car are explained by its engine, wheels, steering, transmission and braking systems, not to forget the seats and the roof for keeping dry. Each of those parts is further explained by the properties of the bits from which it is made, and they from their materials, and the materials by their molecules, and the molecules by their atoms, and they by their subatomic particles... et cetera. We do not know where it ends. A car cannot do anything its parts do not permit, and they in turn are constrained by their molecules etc. Even though a car does nothing its molecules cannot do themselves (speed up, slow down), the unique structure of the car allows us to manipulate the laws of thermodynamics to achieve an outcome that would be vanishingly unlikely if its molecules were not in that particular configuration. For example, there is no thermodynamic law that says humans can't travel 480km in four hours, it is just exceedingly unlikely without a strong tail wind, a big hill or a car. By using energy (increasing entropy), the machine called a car works against the thermodynamic gradient to achieve what, at first glance, is an impossible outcome.

Similarly, there is no reason why H_2O and CO_2 molecules in the air should not combine randomly to form sucrose molecules, it is just exceedingly unlikely. However, given the particular structure of that clever little machine called a chloroplast, molecules of H_2O and CO_2 can be brought into close proximity such that they can utilize ambient solar energy to build the complex sugar molecules which the plant then uses to lift its leaves closer to the sun and, finally, to reproduce itself. Again, the matter-energy pathways for this process are understood in great detail; that is the goal of reductionism, to reduce a complex machine to its most minute properties in order to show exactly how it does just what it does and nothing else. A leaf in the sun cannot produce vanilla icecream just because those particular pathways are not represented in its biochemical pathways.

All of this you have learned in much greater detail than was available to students of my generation, but the principle of reductionism hasn't changed one iota. It is part and parcel of our perception of the universe, something we have accepted with every breath of air for longer than we can remember. If there is one thing we can do that chimps can't, it is that we understand that every big thing is made of little things which work in harmony to produce its outcome. So of course none of our teachers ever explained that they were teaching the particular ontological approach to life, the universe *and* everything called "reductionism," because they weren't told about it either: fish don't know they live in water. So maybe for the first time in your life, you are hearing this explicitly stated: "As a medical student, you were trained in, and totally submerged in, biological reductionism from the moment you entered school. Congratulations, it is probably the most successful intellectual program in human history. It has brought you GPS satellites that can guide a drone to drop a tactical nuclear weapon on you in a thunderstorm at night with an accuracy of millimeters in a thousand kilometers. What more could you ask?"

Well, you could ask this: does biological reductionism explain mental disorder? With a warm, caring smile, your professor will say, "Yes, Virginia, of course it does. We have fMRI scanners and genome assays and probes and radioimmunoassay to detect chemical imbalances, they tell us all we need to know about brain disorders." Reassured, you go off for tea but something isn't quite right. Next day, you approach him again. "Can you tell me," you ask hesitantly, "the name of the model of mental disorder you use in your daily practice, your teaching and your research, which allows you to say that biological reductionism will tell us all we need to know about mental disorder with no unexplained bits left over?" Your professor will look at you uncertainly, then a frisson of perplexity will cross his normally urbane features. With a quick glance around, he will mutter: "I don't know what you mean," and scurry off. (If you want to know, that response came from an eminent professor from Harvard who is heavily involved in DSM-5).

Does the theory of biological reductionism explain mental disorder? That is to say, can we formulate a general statement of an "*unseen causative mechanism* which is *one dimension removed* from the observations...*" of mental disturbance in terms of the matter and energy of the brain? Agreed, biological reductionism explains the fluid retention of acute glomerulo-nephritis very well. We are closing in on some of the mechanisms of cancer and the function of the HIV, but can reductionism also explain the phenomena of mental disorder by reducing them to matters of chemistry? If so, what would a model of mental disorder look like? The unspoken assumption in psychiatry is that biological reductionism is the correct theoretical stance, so therefore a model of mental disorder will not differ substantially from a model of acute glomerulo-nephritis; only a few minor details have to be amended to shift the focus from nephrons to neurons. That is to say, can we reduce the products of the human mind to questions of the properties of molecules? For example, can the enjoyment of poetry or the distress of grief be fully explained as properties of the physical structure and function of the brain? I don't believe they can, and no orthodox biological psychiatrist has ever shown that they can. Worse still, no orthodox biological psychiatrist has ever shown the slightest awareness that this might actually be a question worth considering. Where there should be a reductionist theory of mental disorder, there is an intellectual void. Therefore, we are forced to accept that the widespread faith in biological reductionism as a theoretical explanation for mental disorder is nothing more than an ideological commitment, because it is not a theory in any accepted sense of the word.

This is very strange, you might say; how could so many highly-educated, charming, cultured, caring and liberal professors be so egregiously wrong in their apprehension of the nature of mental disorder? This is not a trivial question. It leads us to another area in the philosophy of science, which is perhaps less a matter of philosophy than the sociology of competitive groups.

***

I'm not sure how science is taught in schools these days but, in my time, we gained the impression that science was a long, wide and straight road leading from the darkness of the Olden Days (i.e. when my parents were younger) into the glorious, sunlit uplands of the Technofuture. Scientists were the wise, caring and rather unworldly creatures who were shepherding humanity along the path to health, wealth and a life of ease. Of course, no teacher would have said as much but this notion was loud and clear. For somebody interested in science, as I was, the future meant studying hard at school in order to get a place in that somewhat mysterious world called "a laboratory." In the late 1960s, when I was studying medicine at university, the molecular biological revolution was in full swing and technology was powering ahead. By the time I began training in psychiatry, the biological juggernaut seemed unstoppable. When our professors stated, as they repeatedly did, that biotechnology was on the verge of delivering the last few secrets of the human mind, we had no reason to doubt them.

Now, decades later, we are no closer than in those halcyon days. If anything, we seem further from a full understanding of the human mind because we now know much more about the incomparable complexity of the brain, and simplistic technologies such as behaviorism have vanished. Meanwhile, the audience of post-modernists in the rear seats keeps up a barrage of catcalls and peanut shells, mocking science as something quite as irrational as politics or sport, indeed, something which is likely to lead to the earth cooking before too long. Science, they say, is no longer the solution to our problems; it is a major part of the problem itself. So who is right?

These problems were not considered widely before 1962, when a small book by an obscure physicist-turned-historian started to attract interest. Thomas Kuhn's aptly named *Structure of Scientific Revolutions* quickly started one. In brief, he argued that the progress of science isn't as clear-cut and straightforward as we might like to think. In fact, it has been punctuated by unpredictable revolutions, during which an old science is abruptly swept away to be replaced by a completely new way of looking at things. His account starts with a period of what he called 'normal science.' Normal science is more or less what you might expect, with collections of scientists in different centers studying their bit of the natural world according to their perception of it. This particular perception or understanding he termed their 'paradigm,' which originally meant the systematic set of all inflections of a word or model. He used it to mean the systematic set of all beliefs about their work. Scientists are trained in a particular paradigm, and their job is to study and research it in order to extend it, thus filling in the gaps so that it becomes complete. This sort of work, which he called 'normal science,' is rather pedestrian and unexciting but it leads steadily toward the goal of a mature science.

Kuhn's historical training, however, showed that scientific reality was never quite as smooth as that ideal. What happened was that, as they beavered away, the scientists came across discrepancies or inconsistencies their model couldn't explain. Most of them simply ignored these little annoyances and pressed on, fairly sure that they would later be explained as perhaps errors in the machines, or exceptions that turned out to support the model. Often, however, the discrepancies didn't go away, but built up until it finally became apparent that the model was in serious trouble. Rather than admit this unpleasant truth, the old guard, who held the reins of power in the laboratories and universities, would fight the complaints vigorously. Then something dramatic happened. Somebody would find something totally unexpected or, more likely, a new interpretation of the data would burst upon the scene and the old model would be shown to be totally inadequate. Within a short time, the old order would be overturned. The old guard would suddenly find themselves shunted to one side as the supporters of the new model raced ahead in demonstrating its remarkable reach and scope. By the time the next generation of students entered the field, they would be taught entirely in the new model and would laugh at the folly of anybody who had been so short-sighted as to think the old one could do anything.

Kuhn used a number of historical examples to demonstrate his point, including the Copernican revolution, the Darwinian period and the change from Newtonian to relativistic physics. He made a number of highly original points that shocked the scientific establishment and provoked a deal of hostility. Firstly, he argued that science isn't as rational as we would like to think. Ignoring discrepancies is not rational, and modifying a model repeatedly to try to incorporate other observations can be silly. During the revolutionary period, the new model would not be able to explain some things as well as the old one, so the choice of one model over another may be no more than the personal preference of the head of the laboratory. Second, he was of the view that the revolutionary period in any field of science would most likely be precipitated by either an outsider or a newcomer. The old guard had been trained in a particular viewpoint, so they were incapable of seeing when it was in trouble, and how. They dismissed its failings as minor quirks which their industrious research would eventually overcome, and were blind to their true significance as fatal anomalies. When a new model was announced, they would fight it bitterly, and Kuhn quoted the great Max Planck who said a scientist could never hope to convince his opponents, he could only wait for them to die. Finally, when the revolution was established, the new generation of scientists would see the world through different eyes and would be unable to understand the old men's point of view. Successive models used in the same field are not just different ways of looking at the same things, they are intellectually incommensurate. Different generations of scientists are not just talking different languages, they live in totally different worlds.

This attempt to summarize Kuhn's life work in one page barely does him a service but it should show why the scientific establishment was outraged by his thesis. Despite the wealth of historical evidence he used, the Grand Old Men of Science were particularly incensed by his view that they didn't have much to contribute to the development of a new field and were, very often, actually obstructive to, if not destructive of, the work of their juniors who were ushering in the millennium. Kuhn's efforts to educate scientists as to the actual conduct of their business were not helped by the post-modernists and various other antagonistic groups who seized on his work as an authoritative vindication of their rabid anti-rational and antiscientific beliefs. Kuhn resented their interpretation of his careful historiographic analysis of the conduct of science but there wasn't much he could do about it. They wanted to believe that "anything goes" in science but refused to accept that his work may, apply equally well to their own, loosely-defined fields as to the more disciplined life in a laboratory. In any event, Thomas Kuhn brought the philosophy of science to the forefront in what we might even call a "Kuhnian revolution in the philosophy of science." We cannot go back to the old view.

For myself, I was soon re-educated in the notion that science is not so rational as its publicists would have us belief. It has its dark side, and scientists themselves are very often far from "wise, caring and rather unworldly creatures shepherding humanity along the path to health, wealth and a life of ease." I have no trouble with this, which is probably very helpful when it comes to dealing with my own specialty, psychiatry. Anybody who takes the longer view of modern psychiatry will be shocked by the elastic way it always seems to include itself on the platform of the sciences, even though its ticket changes every generation or so. Once, you had to be a psychoanalyst to gain entry to the palaces of science, then it was behaviorism but now, it is biological psychiatry. Biopsychiatry's cheerleaders parade around the country with drums and whistles (mostly paid by the drug industry), keeping up a mesmerizing barrage of claims, testimonials and seminars in an endless flood of TV and press "infomercials" that alternately terrify and inspire the general public into believing that, look out, you or your children may be next but don't worry, here comes biopsychiatry to the rescue.

It is all rubbish.

It is the case that, by any rational process of analysis, orthodox psychiatry fails to meet the minimal criteria for a science. It has no agreed, articulated model of its field of mental disorder, and not even a whisper of agreement as to what actually constitutes its field. It lurches from crisis to crisis, the latest being the vast and systematic corruption of academic psychiatry by the drug industry. The psychiatric publishing industry is both corrupt and incompetent, a prisoner of its own myths, while the general public sees only a profession that can't make up its mind about anything except that everybody is mentally ill and need lots of expensive drugs. It is also the case that, by any measure, psychiatry is ripe for a Kuhnian revolution but the establishment seems to have been alerted as they are redoubling their efforts to make sure that no hint of dissatisfaction reaches the ears of medical students and trainees. Which is just as Kuhn predicted.

Chapter 5: Ethics as a Postscript

Ethics has been defined as "the philosophical study of the moral value of human conduct and of the rules and principles that ought to govern it; a social, religious or civil code of behavior considered correct, especially that of a particular group, profession or individual..." In practice, ethics comes down to the set of rules we *ought* to follow. They are not rules of the type: "If you want to survive, you must eat and drink and breathe." That is, we are bound by the same set of survival rules as all other animals. By following the various biological imperatives, we can stay alive and reproduce and probably even prosper. However, there is a different class of rules which other animals do not share, the rules of good conduct. Traditionally, the concept of what constitutes a good or moral life has been regarded as the province of the religious but, in fact, it is an ancient preoccupation and long precedes all the major religions. They simply made a grab for it, anchoring their particular point of view to the Absolute, which meant they were then able to deal with heretics in decidedly unethical ways.

Today, we recognize different branches of the study of moral matters (and I admit I have trouble seeing them as separate). Our friends at Wikipedia divide the field thus:

Meta-ethics is concerned with the theoretical meaning and reference of moral propositions and how their truth values (if any) may be determined;

Normative ethics looks at the practical means of determining a moral course of action;

Applied ethics is about how moral outcomes can be achieved in specific disciplines or situations;

Moral psychology examines how moral capacity or moral agency develops from infancy and its nature; and

Descriptive ethics looks at the moral values people actually follow, regardless of what they claim.

It must not be forgotten that ethics goes beyond the law. The set of civil laws governing citizens is more or less the minimum needed to keep society grumbling along without too many casualties. Ethics or morality extends the scope of rule-governed behavior beyond the limit of "don't get caught." The principle is to give each individual a set of rules that can cover most, if not all, potential conflicts, with the goal of maximizing human welfare. Which leads directly to one of the major questions in modern ethics: how can we justify an anthropocentric ethical system? What should be the starting point in any ethical system? Bear in mind that whatever imperative you choose as The Most Basic Law of Life, somebody else will object to it. For those who no longer accept a divine authority, and given that it is not possible to derive "ought" conclusions from "is" premises, what is the initiating principle for a system of "oughts"? That is, we cannot take any single fact of the world as it exists as the basis for a system of moral rules. Conversely, as the ancient dispute over the geocentric universe showed, ethical beliefs cannot be used to determine our perception of the universe and our place in it. This does seem to leave us in a sticky position: we want a system of "oughts" or rules to control our lives but the only source outside ourselves (divinity) is ruled out of consideration by the doctrine of materialism.

So where do we start? My suggestion is that we start from the position that, so far as we know, earth is the only planet in the universe with life forms. Therefore, we must never do anything to endanger that fact. We do not have the right to push any species into extinction, i.e. we ought not to do that, but there is nobody but posterity to judge us, and even that's not guaranteed. This leads to a restricted form of morality; the rest, about living together, is purely contractual. That is, don't murder or steal because it causes trouble and so on. If anybody can do better than that, I'd be pleased to hear it.

I will admit that I find ethical deliberations overwhelmingly complicated. Nothing is ever as simple as it seems. Debating the nature of mind is much simpler than debating the death sentence or whether animals have rights. This does not suggest it is of no interest but it does say that anybody who thinks ethics is a pushover is either profoundly wrong, or a fanatic (or both).

Scientific ethics is a growth industry, not the least because there is so much dirt for it to grow in. Whereas once, a scientist could do more or less what he (note that) pleased, these days, it is hardly possible to turn around in one's chair without breaching some ethical rule or other, or offending some group of the self-righteous. Ethical rules in science have moved beyond the basics, such as don't chew gum you've left overnight on the lab bench, and don't flick gooballs at the girl on the next bench. These days, every aspect of the work has to be considered for its ethical dimension. Were the rats that are about to donate their livers raised in approved, draft-free housing? Were the test-tubes packed in a sweatshop by political prisoners in a dictatorship? Do we have the right to retain specimens from autopsies because they will help teach medical students? Who has provided support for this experiment and was box 12 on page 95 of the research protocol correctly ticked? Could this experiment provide the basis for a new weapon of mass destruction? There is no end to the ethical considerations, but one question that should not forgotten is "Why?" Are these real considerations or are they simply there to keep some ideologue happy? Are things better than they used to be, or is it just another example of science becoming hostage to pressure groups who decline to accept that there are limits to their behavior, too? Has anybody given any thought to the ultimate goal of the increasing thickets of ethical rules, or will it be like tax law, where each year's crop of new laws is simply added to last year's, which benefits tax lawyers, accountants and tax evaders but not conscientious citizens.

Having said that, it is remarkable that, in psychiatry, ethical standards appear to have slipped very badly in the past few years. Granted, psychiatry has a pretty grim history when it comes to ethics, as Robert Whitaker's *Mad in America* describes in frightening detail, but we would like things to have improved since then. This does not appear to have happened. Whereas once people were locked in ghastly mental hospitals and submitted against their will to various forms of shock therapy and brain surgery, now they must go through a semi-judicial hearing before they can be detained, with lawyers on each side arguing the toss before a tribunal which, at the end, will lock them in a ghastly mental hospital anyway and may give them shock treatment. Today's mental patients are generally not submitted to brain surgery; instead, they are sedated to the point of stupefaction with large doses of very powerful, toxic psychotropic drugs. Moreover, once drugs are started, it is unlikely they will ever be stopped: a person who objects to the drugs will find his dosage increased due to his lack of insight and his threatening behavior.

All this is in the total absence of anything like a formal, articulated model of mental disorder to guide the daily practice of psychiatry, its teaching and its research program. Unfortunately, orthodox psychiatry seems oblivious to this little fact, gleefully spreading the word by all means available that they have mental disorder cornered. That is one part of their publicity program. The other part, as mentioned above, is an unremitting propaganda barrage to terrify the general population into believing that any and every deviation from some undefined standard of psychological perfection is a catastrophe in the making which can only be averted by "seeing your doctor," i.e. taking more and more of those very powerful, toxic drugs for longer and longer. This is especially the case when it comes to children: parents can be frightened into almost anything if it involves their children's futures. In a society that lacks nothing and believes nothing, fear becomes the only ideology capable of mobilizing the masses.

To my admittedly narrow way of thinking, there is something profoundly unethical in all this activity. Telling people that we know for certain what is happening inside their heads, and that we can rectify it before it gets worse, without having prior access to an agreed, declared and properly articulated model of mental disorder, is unethical. I am all too aware that there is nothing in that vast but largely unwritten textbook of scientific ethics that says psychiatrists ought not to make a claim of this nature without a clear statement of the scientific model in use, but that is beside the point. The point is that, while scientific ethics is vague, amorphous and largely inchoate, it is still a reality. The general position is simple: When in doubt, don't. In any field of ethics, it is not the case that, if something isn't actually prohibited, then it is permitted because ethics recognizes that a complete set of moral rules to cover all contingencies is an impossibility. We therefore strive to equip people with the next best thing, a general sense of right and wrong, of what is fair and reasonable or what is sailing a bit too close to the wind. That's all we have. It's probably all we can ever have. Scientists must take responsibility and be accountable for their actions in a transparent system. Anything less and we slide into anarchy or autarchy.

The problem at present is that, in psychiatry, we now have very much less than "responsibility and accountability in a transparent system." We have the appalling spectacle of some of the most powerful and influential members of the psychiatric community peddling their reputations to the highest bidder for secret cash payments. A widely used textbook of basic psychiatry for medical students and general practitioners, *Recognition and Treatment of Psychiatric Disorders: A Psychopharmacology Handbook for Primary Care* by Alan Schatzberg (sometime president of the American Psychiatric Association) and Charles Nemeroff (former head of department at Emory University and close friend of the director of the NIMH, Thomas Insel), was almost entirely ghost-written by people employed by the drug industry. Ghostwriting of important research papers, selective publication of results with suppression of unfavorable studies, favorable publicity in the guise of education in return for secret payments of millions of dollars, these are now the norm.

The US Senate inquiry chaired by Sen. Charles Grassley found that three senior Harvard psychiatrists, Joseph Biederman, Timothy Wilens and Thomas Spencer, failed to declare millions of dollars of drug company money that they had received after they advocated the strongest possible favorable position on prescribing psychiatric drugs to children. In essence, they set the de facto standard that withholding drugs from children was grossly negligent. They were not alone. Former director of NIMH and author of a widely used textbook of psychiatry, Frederick Goodwin, was on the drug companies' payroll, as were psychiatrists Martin Keller of Brown University and Melissa DelBello of Cincinnati University. Drs John Rush and Karen Wagner of University of Texas also received illicit payments, as well as many others.

However, the most egregious penetration of the psychiatric profession by partisan interests is in the committees rewriting the Diagnostic and Statistical Manual for the American Psychiatric Association, where a frightening proportion of committee members have very extensive ties to the drug industry. A 2006 study from Boston showed that "56% of the 170 psychiatrists who worked on the 1994 edition of the DSM-IV had at least one monetary relationship with a drug maker." The study also found that *every one* of the 'experts' on *DSM-IV* panels overseeing 'mood disorders' (which includes depression) and 'schizophrenia/psychotic disorders' had undisclosed financial ties to drug companies. At the time, international sales of drugs to 'treat' these conditions were more than $34 billion" (it is now very much more). This is not just in the US, but is world-wide. Here in Australia, a recently-formed committee to advise the Federal minister for mental health on ADHD consisted almost exclusively of people with long and close ties to the drug industry or their apologists (it has since been disbanded just because of those ties, but only after the community had made a fuss; the minister certainly didn't care). The point of greatest concern is that the minister could not have known whether he was being fed a diet of purified and carefully monitored propaganda for and on behalf of the drug industry, because his "experts" had a clear financial incentive to make sure he never found out.

Granted, none or very little of this is actually illegal but, by the same token, none of it is actually proper. As we used to say, it isn't cricket. The whole point is that mature, responsible people don't need to have the rules of decorum spelled out in infinite detail because an honorable person (a gentleman, as we are no longer allowed to say) knows intuitively where the lines of decent behavior lie (ladies operated so far inside the rules of decency that they were never tempted). Times have changed; there has been a seismic shift in public morality, away from a few rather elementary laws combined with a vaguely-defined but powerful sense of right and wrong, to a bewildering set of laws that nobody understands coupled with the suspension of private morality. With predictable alacrity, a few members of the profession have stepped into this moral vacuum and cheerfully capitalized on what they saw as a golden opportunity to enrich themselves under cover of their colleagues' gullibility. From my very old-fashioned point of view, I see this sort of behavior as psychopathic. I appreciate that full professors at prestigious institutions (who, according to evidence deposed at the Senate enquiry by Professor Biederman of Harvard Medical School, stand one step below the Almighty Herself in the cosmic order of things) may object to the word 'psychopathic' appearing in the same sentence as their names but it is a case of "If the cap fits, then wear it." They were the ones who redefined psychopathy as Antisocial Personality Disorder, so that it applies only to poorly-educated young men, thereby carefully excluding suave and sophisticated criminal manipulators like Bernard Madoff, Sonja Kohn, Ken Lay and Tom Delay – and some well-known psychiatrists who are on the take.

It is my view that all this stems from the demonstrated fact that psychiatry does not have a formal model of mental disorder as the defining element in its practice, teaching and research. This is not just ludicrous but unethical: at present, the profession is spending perhaps hundreds of millions of dollars trying to write a successor to the seriously flawed DSM-IV (be aware of that figure: a lot of these people are university staff, who are paid whether they are on site or not; the APA is not paying that money but the nation is). So far, every indicator is that the flaws in DSM-IV will not only be carried over to the new edition but will be exaggerated by psychiatry's rush to present itself as a science. The time and money now being spent on trying to write a nosology for a non-science should be spent on sorting out the nature of mental disorder and finding a suitable model. Anything less is unethical.

As I have said, these are not minor considerations: we need rules just because having few or none allows people to act selfishly. If there are not clearly defined ethical or moral rules of scientific conduct, then anything goes, which is completely unacceptable. If you want to know why it is unacceptable, look at your children and ask if you would like them to be used in medical experiments against your and their wishes. Yes, that is just utilitarianism again, but let's consider some examples of when that actually happened. During World War II, both the Nazi and Japanese governments conducted vile procedures on captive populations under the pretext of "medical experiments." The

Nazi investigations were conducted on prisoners, both civilian and, especially, Soviet military prisoners of war. Post-war, the major offenders were tried in the notorious "Doctors' trials" at Nuremberg in 1946-47, and a considerable number of them were hanged. The results of their "experiments" were embargoed in perpetuity through respect for their unknown victims.

The Imperial Japanese program in chemical and biological warfare has had much less publicity but it was equally as extensive and as well-organized as the German efforts. Based in north China, it conducted industrial scale experiments on a variety of weapons of mass destruction of very limited use in military settings, but which would have been very effective against civilian populations. These ranged from the simple (testing flame throwers on live prisoners tied to posts, effects of different kinds of grenade explosions on people, and so on) to testing and manufacturing biological weapons using virulent bubonic plague, anthrax, cholera and typhoid organisms. All of these weapons were tested on civilians who had simply been rounded up for the purpose. There were many other grotesque procedures performed on civilian and military prisoners, especially by the innocuous-sounding Unit 731 which was based in north-east China. There are conflicting reports as to the numbers of people murdered during their studies, but certainly not less than 10,000, while up to 600,000 people may have subsequently died as a result of chemical and other weapons developed by this unit. Post-war, only the former Soviet Union prosecuted Japanese scientists who had served in this unit; those in the Allied zone were largely absorbed by industry and academia for their particular skills. These were not amateurs: they were highly-trained and inventive scientists using their knowledge to destroy life – and to advance theirs.

At the same time as this was happening, there was a smaller-scale experiment taking place in the US state of Alabama in which a cohort of some 400 black men who had contracted syphilis were denied treatment until they died. The Tuskegee syphilis experiment began in 1932 and ran until it was finally closed in 1972, a good 25 years after penicillin became readily available for treating syphilis. The men were mostly poor and uneducated rural laborers who were brought into a government-sponsored prospective program to study the long-term effects of syphilis. The devastating effects of syphilis had long been known. During the nineteenth century, it was the commonest cause of admission to mental hospitals (and is the source of the myth that lunatics believe they are Napoleon). Because there was no treatment until the 1920s, it inevitably resulted in a slow and grotesque death. Early forms of treatment included the dangerous mercurial and arsenical drugs as well as the (now) bizarre procedure of infecting patients suffering tertiary (cerebral) syphilis with malaria to induce high fevers, as the organism is especially delicate and dies with high temperatures. For this discovery, the Austrian neurologist Julius Wagner-Juaregg won the 1927 Nobel prize.

When the Tuskegee experiment began, there was essentially no treatment available for the condition, so watching people while the disease took its course was probably not much different from giving people with cancers morphine and making them comfortable. However, that is not the same as actively withholding from them the information that they had this terrible disease (most of them were not single, and were having children) and then denying them access to what was already known to be a cheap and singularly effective treatment, penicillin. The program was supported throughout by the US Public Health Service and information about it was carefully controlled in case it led to the experiment being stopped. In 1966, a young social worker, Peter Buxtun, was assigned to a study of venereal diseases and came across the program. He wrote to the director of the PHS Division of Venereal Diseases, questioning the morality of the research, and was told it had to proceed. After six years of hitting blank walls, he went to the press and the news was made public in July, 1972, after which the program stopped abruptly. The survivors and their relatives were treated and awarded small compensation. It would be easy to say that this was just a typical part of the racist social structure but it wasn't. Several of the medical staff involved were black themselves, and several white members had resigned as they disagreed with it. One of the most important figures in the whole program was a black nurse, Eunice Rivers, who was the local coordinator of the entire research effort and was the only member of staff to stay from inception to closure. Without her very close knowledge of the men and their surroundings, the experiment may have closed earlier.

Recently, a researcher found evidence of a similar experiment in Guatemala in 1946-48, in which almost 700 people, almost all of them men, were deliberately infected with syphilis in order to test the efficacy of penicillin. This was a program involving US and Guatemalan health officials and medical staff, paid by the US PHS Division of Venereal Diseases. The experimental design was simplicity itself: infected prostitutes were taken into prisons, mental hospitals and army barracks. Once infected, the men were treated with antibiotics but nobody knows if they were all treated or what happened to them later.

So what? There have to be a few sacrifices for the greater good, you can't make an omelet without breaking some eggs, there weren't any laws against it then, morality is a private issue, and so on. All this is true, but there is a huge gap between whatever is specifically prohibited by the law, and what is proper. While there will always be arguments over what is or is not frowned upon morally, there is a good test to apply in cases of doubt. It is called the "nearest and dearest" test and it relies on an innate sense of morality which, I would be the first to agree, is probably not a strong basis for judging actions but is still much better than nothing. If there is any doubt as to whether an action is morally correct, just imagine this. Imagine the subject were the person who is nearest and dearest to you: would you still want the experiment or treatment to go ahead? Would you like it for yourself? Would the doctors in the Tuskegee experiment have wanted their wives infected with syphilis? Would any of the politicians who approved the budget have volunteered their children? Don't answer.

We can reverse this little test for those cases where there is some doubt as to the morality of an action which is likely to bring you a large profit, as in the matter of the worthy professors Biederman, Schatzberg, Nemeroff and all the others. If they weren't sure whether it was reasonable to get so much money and hide it, imagine if the psychiatric researcher they loathed and despised most in the world had done it but, for some reason, they never could their own hands on the loot. What would they have said? Would they have just shrugged and got on with their business, or would they have wanted his head on a pike by the university gate? They needn't answer, on the basis that they may incriminate themselves.

The same goes for the universities which had had ample warning that some of their most senior staff were creaming money improperly. They did nothing. Why did they do nothing? Because universities take a large chunk of any incoming research grants for "administrative purposes," rarely less than 50% and often more. An active researcher can pull in tens of millions a year in grants. Universities are expensive businesses, they have big bills. Why should they look closely at all the money sloshing through the spigots into their endowments? Because they should. That's what moral means. It means drawing a very clear line between behavior which meets all the rules, even unstated or implicit rules, and behavior which is just a little bit dickey.

* * *

The principle behind morality is not that it will get you a good seat in heaven or at the best restaurants in town, or that you can use it to club your opponents, but that it fills the gaps between behavior that is prohibited by public law and behavior that is right and proper. We cannot legislate for all contingencies; people have to be responsible and decide each case on its merits. Morality means *not* "closing an eye," it means taking unpleasant decisions, losing an advantage, maybe even losing a battle but still knowing that what you did was correct. I admit that, in these days of monstrous corruption in the public and financial worlds, that's probably a bit cute but anything less leads to chaos (such as we are currently experiencing). In times of chaos, it isn't the powerful and the wealthy and the well-connected who get trampled, it's the weak and poor and marginalized. If you would rather be one of the wealthy and well-connected powerful then please, go and get another job. We don't want you in medicine. If you are such a weak and pathetic character that you need to cream millions of dollars into your hidden accounts and walk around telling people that you are next to God, then you're in the wrong job. Maybe you should even be taking some of those antipsychotic tablets you were so keen for other people to take. Probably, you should just grow a moral sense.

Glossary

Some definitions and explanations to help you find your way through the thickets of philosophical jargon. Please remember that every attempt to define a concept in philosophy immediately provokes a guerrilla campaign by somebody who disagrees with it.

Animism: this is probably the primeval religion, the notion that if humans have something inside them that makes them tick, then everything else must have one, too. However, all the various nymphs, spirits and sprites are often a bit naughty and have to be placated. Gods have to kept quiet with sacrifices (human and otherwise) and some people can learn to tap the universal magic for their own purposes: good magic for shaman-healers, and black for witches and diabolists.

A posteriori: Looking backward; it means to reach a decision after an event. *A posteriori* reasoning is to work backwards from established facts to establish causes.

A priori: Looking forward; it means to reason forward without facts and reach a general conclusion based on what are called 'first principles.'

Ab initio: From the beginning, from the outset.

Behaviorism: the dominant theory of psychology throughout the twentieth century. It was based on the need to eliminate any and all talk of minds from science just because minds are unobservable in principle, and therefore cannot form the basis of a science of human conduct. The major assumption is that the mind can be treated as a "black box," whose inner workings we can never know but which don't concern the scientist. All we need to know is the input (stimulus, environmental contingencies etc) and, by studying the output, we can determine the rules relating input to output in all possible circumstances. It was expected that this would lead to a full understanding of the general rules of behavior and thence to a science which allows us to predict and control all aspects of human behavior. Clearly, early behaviorists expected that there wouldn't be very many rules otherwise their interactions would multiply exponentially and we would never be able to sort them out. They expected that the whole of human behavior would reduce to a small set of general rules which were common to most, if not all, higher animals. This included speech and all other complex behavioral systems.

Behaviorism treated the mind as a "*tabula rasa*," an "empty slate" on which experience writes the precise rules for that person's behavior in accordance with the generic laws of behavior for all organisms. It did not accept any innate drives on the basis that all behavior was learned and therefore could be manipulated. Two variants: Classical, or Pavlovian conditioning theory; and Operant or Skinnerian conditioning theory. Both of these have now been accepted as non-scientific. This caused some consternation in the psychologists' camps as they have had a good century abusing psychiatrists for the non-scientific mentalism of psychoanalysis, except that psychiatrists have now abandoned psychoanalysis and taken up biological psychiatry, which is "more scientific than thou." Psychologists have retaliated by devising "cognitive-behavioral therapy," which hopes to have the best of both worlds. It is, of course, a solecism.

Cognitive bias: see cognitive psychology.

Cognitive dissonance: see cognitive psychology

Cognitive psychology: a psychology which accepts that mental events of some sort occur, and are important in determining behavior. If a person finds his way around a city, it is because he has a mental representation of the city in his head to guide his feet. If a person is distressed, it is because there is "*cognitive dissonance*" between his plans and ambitions and the reality in which he lives, which is experienced as distress. Mental disorder is real, in this model, and is treated by bringing the person's perceptions of the world, and of himself, and his role in the world, into order with reality. Eliminating cognitive dissonance allows the person to achieve his full potential.

In its least sophisticated form, cognitive psychology is indistinguishable from the notion of a *homunculus* in the head. Unfortunately, nobody has found a way of separating the unsophisticated cognitive approach from the sophisticated. The homunculus leads inevitably to an *infinite regress*. There is a way around this problem but ordinary cognitive psychology (say, of Beck's school) hasn't found it yet.

Cognitive bias is the bias introduced by our cognitive apparatus. For example, we are physiologically attuned to detect movement in our environment and we always look at novel movements. We detect patterns (of sound, vision, etc) and respond to them selectively. We expect certain things and this influences what we see around us. We expect our friends and relatives to be well-behaved so we overlook their bad behavior. Similarly, we ignore the good things our enemies do and remember only the bad bits. Humans are biased to detect and remember dangerous or threatening things around them and this shapes their perception of their environments and their lives.

Criticism: analyzing an argument, case, model or theory in order to see whether it is consistent. All scientific progress depends upon criticism of the status quo; it is the fundamental duty, and one of the distinguishing characteristics, of a scientist to criticize his own beliefs. Suppression of criticism is a hallmark of non-science, such as religion or politics. Suppression of criticism is the equal most serious ethical breach of a scientist, the other being forging results.

Cynicism: the habitual tendency to see hidden, base motives as the driving force behind all behavior. The cynic doesn't see any good in people around him, only self-interest; even noble behavior has an ulterior motive (this was the basis of Kissinger's

Grand Diplomacy, that nations act only in self-interested ways and are therefore predictable).

Deduction: a form of reasoning in which conclusions are drawn from given facts, or premises. The conclusion is inherent in the premises and only one conclusion is possible.

Demarcation criterion: a term introduced by the philosopher of science, Karl Popper, to indicate a general test or marker which would allow us to distinguish reliably between science and non-science. Popper said that the concept of irrefutability was the criterion which most reliably demarcated science and metaphysics. Any scientific statement can be proven wrong just by observing the real world whereas metaphysical statements can never be proven wrong. In theory, this restricts the field of science but nobody has ever reached its limits, nor do we expect to run out of scientific topics for a long time. Also, his concept is of limited value early in the development of a field: rigidly applied, it would bar us from considering theories which go beyond the available technology, but new technologies often can derive only from bold theories which transcend the boundaries of current scientific thinking.

Dualism: the notion that there are two separate orders of being in the universe which we must reconcile if we wish to see the universe as a rational or rule-abiding place. One order of being which appears in almost all ontological systems is the ordinary, everyday world of matter and energy in which we live and work. Matter and energy constitute the material or natural order of being or realm (a realm is a region subject to a single rule of law; the natural realm is subject to the rule of natural laws, meaning the time-space continuum). However, all cultures recognize matters of human importance which are manifestly not of the material or natural realm, including all abstract concepts (numbers, beauty, good and evil etc) and unseen entities which are composed of something other than matter and energy (spirit-stuff). These include supernatural beings, including divinities, but it also includes the question of the nature of mind. The behaviorist experiment showed that we cannot devise a science of human conduct which excludes a mental life, but we have never been able to give an account of mind within the framework of materialist science.

Is the human mind of the same order of nature as brick walls and frogs, or is it different? Dualism itself says only that there are two orders of being but it does not specify their origin or nature. *Natural dualism* says that the mind is a natural product of the world as it exists, specifically a product of the brain. *Substance dualism* says that mind and body are both real things but are of different and incommensurable orders of nature. It does not imply magic properties such as immortality. *Property dualism* says that a physical thing or being can have various properties which are not physical in any sense of the term but which are nonetheless real. *Supernatural dualism* says there are entities in the universe which are not part of the material realm of matter and energy, yet they can still interfere in the natural world. See also *monism*.

Eliminative materialism: see materialism.

Emergentism: the notion that, as a physical entity increases in complexity, new properties emerge, which are themselves of higher or lower status. Some authors argue that emergent properties are unpredictable, that we cannot predict them just by looking at the physical machine itself. Others say emergent properties are a predictable outcome of the physical nature of the machine, i.e. they are natural and we can plan for them. Emergent properties are still driven by matter-energy transfers in the machine which we can understand in detail, even if they were unexpected, so the idea of unpredictable emergent properties starts to sound a bit mystical. The real interest in emergentism is whether it could account for the human mind 'emerging' from the brain just because it has reached a particular level of complexity. Could we then build our own intelligent machines?

Empirical, empiricism: a product of experience. An empirical fact is a fact gained by experience of the real world. Empiricism is a particular form of psychological philosophy or epistemology which says that all our knowledge comes ultimately from experience of the real world. All concepts and beliefs must, in the final analysis, derive from and be related to actual experiences; an extreme empiricist would argue that there are no true abstract concepts.

Epiphenomenalism: the notion that certain properties play no part in the causation of the machine's performance. The report of a rifle does not speed the bullet forward but is an end result of the explosion of the charge that propelled the bullet. Pain does not cause appendicitis, but is an end result of the inflammatory process. The classic quote is from Thomas Huxley, who said the mind is no more causative of events in the brain than the cloud of steam over a factory controls what happens on its floor.

Epistemology: from Gk. *episteme* – knowledge, and *logos* – the word or explanation. This is the study of the conditions and nature of knowledge as we apprehend it. It concerns the process and form of knowledge, not the content, so it looks at what it takes for something to be a belief, or a falsehood, or how we can know anything and what permits us to accept a proposition as truth etc. There are different kinds of knowledge such as propositional knowledge, empirical and deductive, etc. A very big and fascinating field.

Folk psychology: Wilhelm Wundt's apt term for the common person's concept of how the human mind works. Essentially, it sees the mind as a smaller version of a person, sitting inside the head, looking out through the eyes and listening to the broadcasts as they are picked up by the ears. This concept sees the mental life as causal of observable behavior. It incorporates everyday notions of truth and falsity, honor and treachery, diligence and laziness, etc. but does not explain them as it has no explanation of mind or mind-body interaction. The mind is a "mere fact." It leads to simple forms of cognitive psychology.

Functionalism: One of the latest theories of mind, an attempt to steer a middle path between the mindlessness of behaviorism and the wild excesses of unrestrained mentalism (which everybody knows to mean psychoanalysis). It is driven very largely by an unrestrained antagonism toward dualism. The functionalist sees a mental state not so much as a state with defined mental properties (i.e. the mental component or property of a mental state is hardly relevant) but as an intervening computational state between the environmental stimulus and the behavioral output. Thus, the bits of the brain that generate this state could be replaced by silicon chips and neither the subject nor his audience would be any the wiser. In its extreme form, it says that full human conscious awareness could be generated in a suitable computer. However, if functionalism is antidualist, it must be a monist theory of mind, which raises all sorts of new difficulties.

Homunculus: a "little man," meaning the idea of a little man inside the head who does all the clever things we need to explain. It is non-scientific because it sets up an *infinite regress.*

Ideology: a unified system of belief which must be accepted as a matter of faith rather than by reason. An ideology is not open to discussion or dispute. The term tends to be reserved for politics, especially the fanatical, all-encompassing, all-explaining historicist types which claim to have discovered "laws" of history, and can therefore make predictions and diagnoses. Religious beliefs are normally known as dogma rather than ideology but the effect is the same. An ideologue is a person who unthinkingly adheres to an ideology; also a person who studies and develops an ideology to the point where other people can see its far-sighted brilliance, especially when encouraged to do so at the point of a gun.

Identity theory: see mind-body identity theory.

Induction: a form of inference in which general conclusions are drawn from an incomplete set of observations or data. It is very much how we run our daily lives but it is not good enough in the search for general truths: anecdotes never add up to a general truth.

Infinite regress: Where did the chicken come from? An egg. And where did the egg come from? A chicken. This explanation goes back and back but it goes nowhere. After hearing it a million times, you will know no more than if you had heard it once. It is a regressive explanation, in that it goes backward (most explanations do) and it is infinite, because it never stops (In fact, in its proper form, it does: the answer to the question of what came first is…. A different sort of chicken).

It is important to be able to recognize an infinite regress as people often use them in cognitive psychology: "And what allows us to find our way around? We have a map-reading facility in our cerebral cortex." This is not an explanation at all, because we now have to explain a map-reading facility. It goes back a long way, to the French author, Moliere, who mocked the physicians of his day: "They ask me why opium causes people to sleep and I tell them it is because of a dormitive principle, a *virtus dormitiva*, and the learned gentlemen nod sagely and are satisfied." He hadn't explained anything, because he would then need to show how a dormitive principle puts people to sleep. This is not the same as a tautology, which is to explain something in terms of itself, such as: "He was scared of the dog because it provoked terror." In grammar, a tautology is to state the same quality twice in different ways: A new innovation (innovation just means new); a regular square. Tautologies are common in psychiatry and psychology: "His sad mood put him in a state of depression" or "And why are you so sad today?" "Oh, it's my depression, it always does it."

Ipso facto: Latin, "by that very fact." "Any person found on these premises is *ipso facto* trespassing." The single fact that you are on the premises proves you are trespassing.

Logic: the study of valid inference, or the study of consistent beliefs. I prefer the former definition because I think it is broader but I won't argue the point. Given a certain lump of information, what conclusions can we justifiably draw? There are different types of logic, with the modern forms all but indistinguishable from mathematics. Computers are logic machines, where *logical operations* are mechanized.

Logical operation: a rule-governed operation or procedure performed upon a proposition or set of propositions to define or transform their relationship. A logical operator is an abstract concept of much the same order as the operators in mathematics (+, -, x, /), except that it transforms the status or relationships of propositions instead of values. There is one unary operator (negation, transforms a single proposition) and a range of binary operators (and, or, implies, not and, not or, etc.) which transform two.

Materialism: the basic set of beliefs underlying western science, namely, that there is nothing in the universe beyond matter and energy and their interactions. This is too restrictive so we now allow: "...beyond matter and energy and *the informational states governing* their interactions." See *science*. Strict materialism denies there is any supernatural element in the universe; a moderate position would be that there may be but we can't study it so we'll never know, i.e. agnosticism. The methods and principles of science can only apply to the realm for which they were intended, i.e. the material realm of matter and energy. See *scientism.*

Eliminative materialism is the belief that advances in the material sciences will eliminate a lot of problems by giving a material explanation for what now seems immaterial. The standard example is the way science eliminated the morning and evening stars by showing that they are, in fact, different appearances of the planet Venus. That's not a good example, because they were not immaterial. A better example is the notion that epilepsy was the manifestation of demonic possession. Medical advances showed it is due to an unstable electric focus in the brain which causes a generalized discharge of all neurons, and this is manifest as the seizure.

Promissory materialism isn't really so different, it says "Don't worry about that problem, science will soon explain it away." The most widespread example is the claim that all mental disorder will soon be shown to be a special case of brain disorder, i.e. science will explain away all mental disorder, and psychiatry will become a subspecialty of neurology. Scientific progress will explain mental disorder as a case of disturbances of matter and energy. The 'promise of science' is that it will eliminate the irrational notion that being mentally-disturbed has anything to do with mental concepts, such as losses or fear of the future.

Metaphysics: beyond physics, essentially meaning those questions which are forever beyond the reach of physics (and all the empirical sciences). So, any question which cannot be resolved by empirical evidence is an example of metaphysics, such as questions of good and evil, the origin of the universe, life after death, and so on. Metaphysics has had a bad press for a long time, partly because of the Platonic notion of the goal of things, or teleology. Animals do not evolve in order to survive, they survive because they fitted an ecological niche, which they then exploited. The goal of men is not to be noble, or warlike, nor is the goal of women to be mothers. We are not drawn to a generic future goal: this notion has done a lot of damage to metaphysics. However, humans can determine an individual goal for themselves and work toward it. It is important to be able to recognize metaphysical questions masquerading as scientific subjects, especially when somebody is claiming that his research program will solve one if only he had some more money. Empirical evidence has no bearing on metaphysical questions.

Mind-brain identity theory: a theory from the 1950s and 60s which tried to solve the problem of mind by claiming that, as a matter of fact, mind and body are identical, i.e. they are one and the same thing, or they are of exactly the same nature, so mind-body interaction is no longer a problem. It led to more problems than it solved and was quietly dropped (or kicked aside by the functionalists) but it pops up from time to time in psychiatry, when people claim that mental disorder just is brain disorder or that the two terms are interchangeable. They are not.

Model: an attempt to make a physical embodiment of the essential principles of a particular theory in order to test it under real conditions. A model is an actual working example of a cut down version of the theory. It emphasizes the theory's major points to facilitate their testing, but at the expense of simplifying the theory and overlooking some of its consequences. For example, given the theory of heavier than air flight, we can build a model aircraft based on the reality of an aerofoil. See *theory*.

Modernism: The world-view of late nineteenth century Western rationalist-imperialist-industrialists etc. It is important not to fall into the error of thinking that modernism was only an artistic fad, of which cubism was a well-known example. The modernist view said that the universe is a rational place, governed by unbending laws which, through the diligent application of our highly-developed and perfectly rational thought processes, we can come to understand in their entirety and thereby manipulate to our advantage. It was essentially a triumphalist viewpoint, Man-as-Colossus standing astride the world, stern yet benign until moved to justified wrath. There was no room for the supernatural in this approach, although a distant and appreciative God could still be worshipped from 11.00 to 12.00 on Sundays, business permitting. This was the shrinking world of explosively-expanding science, business, commerce, conquest and pomposity, exemplified in Elgar's Pomp and Circumstance Marches. It climaxed in World War I and thereafter ran out of puff about as fast as the *Hindenburg*. Today, it survives in attenuated form in, you got it, economics. See Post-Modernism.

Monism: the opposite of dualism, i.e. the notion that there is only one order of being in the universe. Monism says that, despite appearances, there is only one reality. A few monists believe that everything is thought, one or two argue that everything is energy while the rest say everything is matter and energy. Ever since Einstein, we do not see the matter-energy duality as a case of dualism, because they both belong to the time-space continuum and are jointly subject to the same laws of physics. A monist explanation of mind says that, despite appearances, mind and body are of one and the same nature. Scientific monism says they both belong to the material realm of matter and energy although nobody has yet worked out how matter and energy give rise to two overtly incommensurable experiences when, mathematically, they are of the same realm.

Occam's Razor: the 'principle of parsimony,' i.e. that the number of explanatory entities must not expand beyond the absolute minimum required to explain the observation in full. Science is lean and elegant, and fripperies will not be tolerated unless they play an essential role in the causation of the events, in which case they aren't just fripperies.

Ontology: the basic statement of one's fundamental understanding of the nature of reality. A *monist* ontology says that there is only one order of being. A *spiritualist* or **supernatural** ontology says that everything is spiritual by nature, that appearances are deceptive. A Manichean ontology sees everything in terms of polar opposites (good and bad, male and female, light and dark, etc) and will attempt to explain appearances in these terms.

Panpsychism: the notion that mental properties or stuff are not unique to humans but are distributed throughout the universe as inherent or immanent properties of matter. A panpsychist says that all atoms have mental attributes but these only amount to a mind when certain conditions prevail (i.e. the matter is assembled in the form of a brain). This does not explain the nature and workings of the mind, it only says where it came from. It is not a scientific theory as there is no conceivable test that could disprove it. Some people try to equate mind with organization, but this achieves nothing as diamonds are highly organized on an atomic level but they are totally inert inside so there can be no mental properties.

Plus ça change, plus c'est la même chose. The more things change, the more they stay the same. Sometimes heroic changes bring us right back to where we started. A tyrannical government is overthrown by revolutionaries, who soon become tyrannical in their own right.

Post-modernism: See modernism. I declare my prejudice: Post-modernism (po-mo to the in-crowd) is absolutely the silliest doctrine ever embraced by avowedly intelligent people, not excluding astral travelling and necromancy. Post-modernism is a justified reaction against the cosmic conceit of the notion that the universe is a small, sensible sort of place that we jolly good chaps can understand with just a bit of effort in between making money, war, good whiskey and good horses. Who ever believed such a thing? I did. When I was a child, I believed everything in the Children's Encyclopedia of Great Scientists, which was passionately modernist in outlook. Since then, we have stopped being quite so conceited. We have some idea that some things in the universe are too complicated for humans to meddle with, while others may in fact be beyond us. We accept that we are full of unstated prejudices, meaning we are not so rational after all. Current post-modernism takes this ball and runs over the nearest cliff with it: There is no such thing as rationalism, all is prejudice; there are no absolutes, everything is relative to the individual's cultural background; there is nothing honorable, everything is done for power and prestige, and so on. That, of course, would include the post-modernists who, oddly enough, seem to believe that their injunctions don't apply to them. The way to deal with a persistent post-modernist (and they are *very* persistent) is to avoid claiming any absolutes. So we may never know everything about the universe? Who cares? There's more than enough to keep us occupied during my lifetime. So the human mind isn't totally rational? I can live with that, but it's rational enough for me to know the difference between a fresh egg and a rotten one.

Pragmatism: a doctrine mainly from the US in the latter part of the nineteenth century. It tries to avoid absolutes and looks at outcomes and processes as the defining features of a statement or claim. Absolute truth cannot be determined because the methods of establishing truth will necessarily bias the process. This doctrine has had a pervasive influence in areas such as law and politics.

Promissory materialism: see materialism.

Property dualism: see dualism.

Rationalism: the idea that life should be lived according to established rational principles and that the universe can be understood as a rational place: "Everything has a cause; nothing happens without good reason." This is a very powerful part of the ontology of materialism and thence of Western science. Our entire understanding of the universe is that it follows rules and that, by a process of ordered inquiry, we can discover and then manipulate those rules to our advantage. Behaviorism was part of the rationalist heritage, the idea that we could reduce all human behavior to a set of non-mentalist principles common to most other animals. At its extreme, it said there is no fundamental difference between humans and other animals. As rationalists, behaviorists needed to see humans as clockwork robots; they could not accept such random factors as a sense of play, curiosity, innate motivation, revenge, etc. The extreme form of rationalism is the modernist illusion, i.e. the notion that we live in a world of infinite potential which, as masters of our own destiny, we can shape to our will (but beware of the law of unintended consequences).

Reductionism: the basis of Western science, this is the notion that the properties or behavior of a high order entity can be explained in their entirety as the outcome of the properties or behavior of the lower order entities from which it is composed. In order to understand something, we take it apart and see how the parts interact. Even though a property may be unexpected, a full knowledge of its parts will always reveal the exact matter-energy equations which allowed that property to appear. Thereby, we can duplicate the property in another machine or improve on it. Within the world of scientists, there is a powerful constituency that argues that a full understanding of the brain's structure will tell us all there is to know about human life. Others argue that there is more to the mind than the brain, that the mind has emergent properties which operate in an irreducible realm just because it involves symbols, and symbols are never reducible to their substrate (otherwise they wouldn't be symbols).

Relativisim: the notion that there are no absolutes, such as truth or validity, in that everything is relative, specifically to the individual's culture and prejudices. Moral relativism says that all moral injunctions are products of and limited to the individual's culture and era, that there are no universal moral imperatives. We live in a sea of shifting values and, if we think there is any certainty, we are deluding ourselves. Including that statement?

Science: the very broad, undirected but rule-governed endeavor directed at understanding the full matter-energy relationships throughout the universe (which means back to the beginning of the universe, however that was). Since it is now agreed that there is more to the observable universe than matter and energy, the definition has been expanded to include the concept of information. Information is now seen as an integral part of the natural world.

Scientism: the inappropriate application of scientific methods and procedures to questions with no empirical content, i.e. trying to solve metaphysical questions by laboratory techniques. Hence, we can speak of biologism, physicalism and historicism.

Skepticism: the systematic refusal to accept the authenticity or validity of accepted beliefs; systematic doubt. Healthy skepticism is part of the scientific tradition, as criticism is the engine of scientific progress. The pathological skeptic refuses to accept anything as true or valid (except his own opinion), and is one of the paranoid variants. Never argue with a pathological skeptic.

Substance dualism: see dualism.

Sui generis: "of its own kind," and thence unique.

Supernatural: above or beyond natural. Essentially, this means any entity or process that breaches the laws of the natural universe. Remember that when Newton formulated the laws of gravity, the concept of action at a distance (which is the essence of the force of gravity) was considered one of the characteristic features of the supernatural, and thus caused Newton considerable anguish before he published his work. This is a little strange, as he was a devout supernaturalist who actually spent a large part of his life pursuing crackpot ideas (he spent another large part locked in vitriolic battles with his competitors). It has sometimes been said of him that he was not so much the first scientist in history as the last magician.

A supernatural entity can suspend, bypass or otherwise interfere with the laws of the natural world. Remember Ambrose Bierce: "Prayer: a plea that the laws of the universe be temporarily annulled in favor of the petitioner, confessedly unworthy."

Tautology: Saying the same thing twice in a different way. This is common in psychology, where people often take an observation to be explained, rephrase it in a different jargon, and then think they have explained it. Skinner did this all the time, his *Beyond Freedom and Dignity* was little more than a tangled mess of tautologies.

Theory: a postulated explanation of observable events which is one dimension removed from the events themselves. The theory causatively joins or links the observations by proposing a rational mechanism by which the preceding event could conceivably give rise to the subsequent event. A theory is a statement of an idea only; some theories are so complex that they exist in mathematical form only. Different observations that comprise a single class of events (e.g. the class of events known as the group of mental disorders) must be united by a single theory. It is not possible to propose a different theory of causation for each one, because they would not then belong to the same class. The number of explanatory entities must not expand beyond the minimal number capable of explaining the events (Occam's razor). The preferred theory is the least complex with the broadest scope. See *model*.

Truism: a proposition that can never be wrong: "Either Elvis is dead or he is alive." Psychiatry and psychology are rife with hidden truisms masquerading as explanations.

References

These are just notes so I won't be giving detailed references. All material mentioned in these chapters is fully referenced in my books, as follow:

McLaren N. *Humanizing Madness: Psychiatry and the Cognitive Neurosciences.* 2007; Ann Arbor, Mi.: Future Psychiatry Press. ISBN 978 1 932690 39 2.

McLaren N. *Humanizing Psychiatry: The Biocognitive Model.* 2009; Ann Arbor, Mi.: Future Psychiatry Press. ISBN 978 1 615990 11 5.

McLaren N. *Humanizing Psychiatrists: Toward a Humane Psychiatry.* Ann Arbor, Mi.: Future Psychiatry Press. 2010 ISBN 978 1 615990 60 3

Other recommended reading:

Gribbin, John (2002): *Science: A history 1543-2001.* Penguin/Allen Lane.

Stumpf Samuel (1993): *Socrates to Sartre: A history of philosophy.* 5th Edition. New York: McGraw Hill.

Whitaker, Robert (2002). *Mad in America: Bad Science, Bad Medicine and the Enduring Mistreatment of the Mentally Ill.* New York: Perseus Books.

Whitaker, Robert (2009). *Anatomy of an Epidemic: Magic Bullets, Psychiatric Drugs and the Astonishing Rise of Mental Illness in America.*

Noam Chomsky maintains a very detailed bibliography at www.chomsky.info. http://www.chomsky.info/articles/1967----.htm "Skinner's *Verbal Behavior*" http://www.chomsky.info/articles/19711230.htm "Skinner's *Beyond Freedom and Dignity*"

These papers are brilliant examples of the devastating intellectual critique. Even if you don't know much about Skinner, they are worth reading.

About the Author

Despite anything you have heard, the author is not an "antipsychiatrist." He is a fully qualified, fully paid up and fully engaged psychiatrist in private practice in Darwin, in Australia's remote north. He is, however, virulently opposed to bad psychiatry, and would not object to being called an "anti-bad-psychiatrist." Practically the whole of psychiatry in the world today is bad. It is, indeed, very bad, and the reason has been established by philosophy. Specifically, psychiatry is not a science just because it fails every known test of what constitutes a science. The question of what constitutes a science is known as the philosophy of science, so philosophers come in handy after all.

Jock McLaren was born in a tiny town in the wheat belt of Western Australia and went to school in a slightly larger town on the far south coast of WA. He studied medicine at the University of WA and then psychiatry, graduating in 1977. He has been in full-time practice ever since, including five years in a Veterans' hospital and six years as the Regional Psychiatrist in WA's remote Kimberley Region, before he moved to Darwin. He lives in the bush out of Darwin with his family and various wild animals, including the family cat. Because there isn't a lot to do in the bush at night, he writes papers and books with a philosophical bent which are uniformly loathed and ignored by the mainstream of psychiatry.

Index

Look for these other great books from Future Psychiatry Press

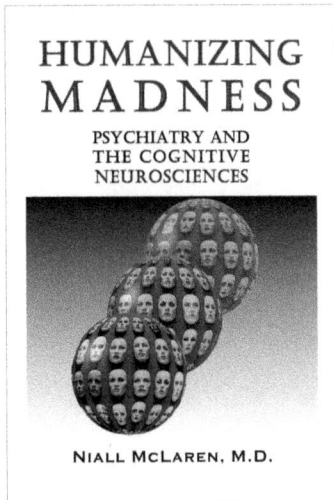

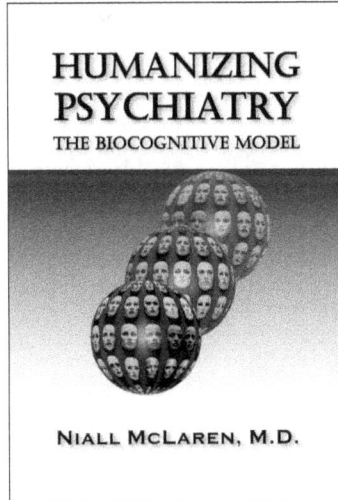

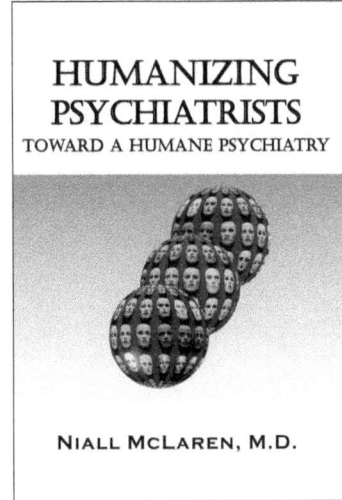

www.ingramcontent.com/pod-product-compliance
Lightning Source LLC
LaVergne TN
LVHW061226060426
835509LV00012B/1447